The Fertility Sourcebook

ALSO BY M. SARA ROSENTHAL:

The Thyroid Sourcebook (Lowell House, 1993)
The Gynecological Sourcebook (Lowell House 1994)
The Pregnancy Sourcebook (Lowell House, 1994)
The Breastfeeding Sourcebook (Lowell House, 1995)

The Fertility Sourcebook

Everything You Need to Know

by

M. Sara Rosenthal

Foreword by

Masood A. Khatamee, M.D., F.A.C.O.G.,
Executive Director, Fertility Research Foundation

Lowell House
Los Angeles

Contemporary Books
Chicago

Library of Congress Cataloging-in-Publication Data

Rosenthal, M. Sara.
  The fertility sourcebook : everything you need to know / by M. Sara Rosenthal ; fore-
word by Masood A. Khatamee.
     p.   cm.
  Includes bibliographical references and index.
  ISBN 1-56565-213-4
  1. Infertility—Popular works.   I. Title.
RC889.R84   1995
616.6'92—dc20   95-2351
                                                                              CIP

Requests for such permissions should be addressed to:
Lowell House
2029 Century Park East, Suite 3290
Los Angeles, CA 90067

Lowell House books can be purchased at special discounts when ordered in bulk
for premiums and special sales. Contact Department VH at the address above.

Publisher: Jack Artenstein
General Manager, Lowell House Adult: Bud Sperry
Text Design: Mary Ballachino / Merrimac Design

Manufactured in the United States of America
10 9 8 7 6 5 4 3 2 1

To my husband

Contents

Acknowledgments

If it weren't for the commitment, hard work, and guidance of the following people, this book would never have been written: Masood A. Khatamee, M.D., F.A.C.O.G., Executive Director of the Fertility Research Foundation, who served as medical advisor; my research assistant, Ellen Tulchinsky, B.A., M.L.I.S.; my editorial assistant, journalist Laura Tulchinsky, B.A.; my editor, Bud Sperry, and my copy editor Dianne Woo.

Special thanks to the physicians and health practitioners who donated their time and expertise: Jerald Bain, M.D., F.R.C.P.(C); Susan R. George, M.D., F.R.C.P. (C), F.A.C.P.; Dianne Hindman, B.Sc., P.H.M.; Keith Jarvi, M.D., F.R.C.S. (C); Matthew Lazar, M.D., F.R.C.P. (C), F.A.C.P; Michelle Long, M.D.; Kelly S. MacDonald, M.D., F.R.C.P. (C); Michael Policar, M.D., F.A.C.O.G.; and Suzanne Pratt, M.D., F.A.C.O.G.

I'd also like to thank Diane Allen, Executive Director of the Toronto Chapter of the Infertility Awareness Association of Canada, who provided me with so many valuable contacts, resources, and materials. Finally, thanks to all of the infertility patients I interviewed. Your stories, struggles, and important suggestions were very much appreciated.

In the moral support department, thanks to my husband, Gary S. Karp, and all the relatives and friends who cheered me on.

Foreword

In the twenty years I've devoted to infertility patients in New York City, it can be safely said that the couples with the most tangible success were those who sought accurate information and thoroughly educated themselves about their conditions and treatment needs. *The Fertility Sourcebook* gives you the proper tools you need to accomplish this goal. The crucial element in achieving successful fertility treatment is carefully choosing the right doctor. The commitment couples make to their skilled clinician, regardless of the treatment's outcome, affects their treatment options. Staying the course with a single practitioner as opposed to "physician hopping" avoids the possibility of gaps in treatment that may lead to important clinical signs being overlooked.

The standard of quality care dictates that a fertility investigation should not exceed a duration of two months, nor should an investigation be halted and treatment commenced as soon as a single factor, such as a cervical factor, is discovered. Couples should be aware of the possibility of "iatrogenic infertility" arising. This occurs when the origin of infertility goes undiscovered as a result of lack of knowledge or interest on the part of the physician, causing procrastination of treatment if not permanent or irreversible infertility related to the physician's mismanagement of the problem.

Infertility specialists are usually devoted to that sole issue, and do not generally diverge into the areas of obstetrics to avoid the obvious distractions that are inherent to these practices. For example, if your physician canceled your post-coital test due to a delivery, it is time to search for another doctor. The time and attention devoted to your individual case is as important as the timing of various clinical tests.

For example, in my own practice, we strongly believe in the consultation, done in the initial visit. Regarded as the most important step in the fertility investigation, this allows the physician the opportunity to take a couple's thorough medical and reproductive histories, as well as allowing time to get to know them and assess their personal needs regarding effective treatment that is right for them as *individuals*. Treatment will take into account their current needs as well as past treatments. It is always important that both partners be present for this crucial visit, preferably at the beginning of the female partner's menstrual cycle. An uninterrupted session lasting from 60-90 minutes should be devoted to this initial interview, while instructions and educational material will lead to more effective treatment.

Generally, no testing is performed at this initial visit unless time constraints and scheduling concerns (as in the case of a patient traveling out of state) make it difficult for the patient to return for a subsequent visit. When scheduling an appointment, it is that important the male pa-tient be advised to abstain from intercourse for at least two days, as the semen analysis would most likely be performed on the first visit. The premise of bringing male patients into the office for testing is, in itself, difficult to achieve, as the majority of male partners encountered hesitate to come with their female partners for evaluation. However, it is an important component of the educational phase of their treatment. Male partners need to have their semen analyzed, discuss the results based on what is visible under the microscope, and if possible, be allowed to view their own specimens under the microscope to enhance their awareness.

For females, a pelvic exam is performed at the first consultation. This usually involves a Pap smear, urine tests, some hormonal testing, as well as screenings for various sexually transmitted diseases and other conditions (such as Rubella), which could pose danger to a potential preg-nancy. Although patient compliance is less than optimal in our less motivated patients, it is also advised that patients take their basal body temperature and bring these charts to each visit. On the day of the initial visit, they are shown how to use the basal temperature thermometer (if they are not acquainted with one), while all of their questions are answered.

The first cycle should be devoted to noninvasive testing, including a postcoital test (PCT), discussed in Chapter 5 of this book. Once the clinical data has been compiled from these prelimi-nary tests, a detailed consultation should then be scheduled with the couple to discuss the results and further treatment options. The second cycle is usually devoted to more invasive diagnostic measures, and condom use is recommended to our patients to avoid possible ill effects of certain tests on undiagnosed early pregnancy.

It is abundantly clear that a fertility investigation—even in the event of endoscopic surgery—should not have a duration of more than two or three months. On the other hand, when a single factor is isolated, and the investigation is halted to begin treatment, precious months may be sacrificed if another factor is overlooked due to an *incomplete* investigation.

Fertility treatment can be lengthy and frustrating. It would seem, at times, that the neces-sary collaboration between specialists prolongs the procurement of the end result. Nevertheless, keep in mind that all treatment must adhere to a reasonable timetable, and the parameters for all modes of therapy must be made clear by your physicians. For instance, if a physician tells you to "take clomiphene citrate for six months and come back if you are not pregnant," it would indi-cate to the well-informed patients that this practitioner is either less than interested in helping you achieve pregnancy, or unschooled in the monitoring and administration of clomiphene cit-rate. It could also indicate that he or she is less than interested in treating infertility. Such an in-stance is cause for concern.

Take care that your testing and analyses, including ultrasound, are *directly* monitored by your physician. It is not in the best interest of the patient to be juggled between various practitioners to obtain testing. For example, in our practice, many tests are performed by our office using an outside facility. This affords us the opportunity to establish that all-important continuity with the patient, as well as to monitor the safety and accuracy of imaging equipment. We also ensure that a certified radiologist is in attendance.

Regarding the issue of Assisted Reproductive Technology (ART), it has sparked a virtual revolution for practitioners, opening up a wellspring of hope for both infertile and sterile couples. New procedures surface almost every month as this new science is advancing exponentially. In many cases, our moral and legal evolution lags behind our scientific evolution. One is hard-pressed to give answers to the many questions that arise concerning inheritance of the offspring, and disclosure issues.

This book provides you with guidelines that will aid you in choosing a reputable ART clinic. Valuable information to consider and questions to ask your health care provider when your are an ART candidate are also provided. Of primary concern is the distinction between the rate of live births and the rate of pregnancies. The latter will always be higher. Always be more concerned with the "baby-take-home" percentage.

Be certain that before considering ART, complete and thorough treatment for infertility conditions has been attempted. Some centers will try to coerce patients into rushing directly into ART treatment before other less costly options have been explored. Stringent medical guidelines governing proper medical and surgical treatment must be adhered to, and patients should beware centers that want hasty decisions regarding ART, as this would be an obvious scheme for monetary gain.

Finally, an issue close to my heart, and held by many physicians as being of paramount importance, is that of *infertility prevention*—also discussed in this book. Twenty percent of North American couples to date are infertile, and the numbers are increasing according to the American College of Obstetrics and Gynecology. This figure accounts for roughly 12 million couples in the United States alone, and more than 58 million couples worldwide. Infertility prevention, as a component of sex education, is not widely addressed.

Infertility is caused mostly by sexually transmitted diseases (STDs), and even in well-educated, industrialized countries, such as the United States and Canada, the medical community is failing to stem the tide of STDs, which lead to infertility. Other causes of infertility are ovarian dysfunction, abnormal sperm physiology and endometriosis. Unfortunately, information about their origins and prevention is grossly lacking. In 1985, I proposed to the medical community that we should endeavor to prevent infertility at all costs. The common-sense modalities we encourage physicians to implement with their patients, have received approval from leading health authorities such as the World Health Organization, the American Medical Association, the American Fertility Society, the American College of Physicians and Surgeons, and the Surgeon General of the United States.

By focusing on infertility prevention, we will be able to help eliminate some of the common, but completely preventable causes of infertility: STDs. Secondly, the success rate for pregnancy in infertility intervention is dismal: a mere 13%. Logically, it is more cost-effective for the medical community to concentrate on prevention rather than treating resulting conditions. Unfortunately, it appears from the low success rates inherent in infertility treatment, that this is the only medical discipline that permits a failure rate of no less than 87%! Prevention must be addressed to ward off further tragedy.

The ramifications of infertility treatment are the tremendous costs involved with investigation and treatment. *Only 1% of infertile couples can afford the expense of Assisted Reproductive Technology. (ART).* At this rate, couples in the United States alone invest over 70 million dollars in procedures that offer only a 13% success rate, according to the United States Congress Office of Technology Assessment 1989 estimate. In addition to the financial burdens this presents, infertility leaves emotional and psychological scars. Relationships erode under the strain, families flounder, and the very fabric of society, the family unit, is undermined.

Currently, while the World Health Organization acknowledges that infertility prevention lags behind treatment, there are some practical suggestions I give my patients regarding prevention. Even if you, personally, cannot practice these measures, pass them on to your friends, relatives, and hopefully . . . children:

1. Women aged 18-28 are optimally fertile. Fertility decreases with passing time, sharply declining at age 35, and by age 40, becoming the exception rather than the rule. ART is substantially less effective after age 38.

2. STDs pose the greatest threat to the reproductive tract in both men and women. Oral contraceptives will prevent pregnancy but not STDs. Condoms should be used at all times.

3. If you've never had children, and would like to, do NOT use an intrauterine device (IUD). IUDs are associated with pelvic infections and subsequent infertility.

4. If you have symptoms of endometriosis (discussed in Chapter 6 of this book), you MUST have a diagnostic laparoscopy to investigate. Women with mothers or sisters afflicted with endometriosis are at high risk. This condition worsens with age, and can lead to infertility.

5. Ovarian dysfunction is being associated with industrial contaminants, and may be aggravated by smoking, drug abuse and pollution. Avoid all "avoidable" toxins! (See chapter 2.)

6. Male subfertility is increasing at alarming rates. In 1960, it was estimated that 6-10% of adult males were subfertile. By 1990, estimates rose to 35-40%. Environmental factors are undoubtedly responsible but more research needs to be done. Be aware, and watch the headlines (see chapter 2).

This book will help an infertile couple seek proper advice and treatment. It will also help to educate you about quality fertility treatment and tell you how to maximize your own fertility. Ultimately, the combination of sound prevention and early treatment will preserve the ability of individuals to procreate in the future, and allow loving couples to raise the dear families they so strongly desire.

Masood A. Khatamee, M.D., F.A.C.O.G.
Associate Clinical Professor, Department of Obstetrics/Gynecology
New York University School of Medicine
New York, New York

Executive Director
Fertility Research Foundation
New York, New York

Introduction
Why *This* Book . . . and Why *Now*?

The inspiration to write *The Fertility Sourcebook* originally came from my own bout with infertility. In light of my experience of not getting pregnant, "losing" friends to pregnancy and parenthood, and suffering rude comments, unwanted advice, and criticism from outsiders, however, I became painfully aware that there was a dearth of information regarding initial conception planning, diagnosis, and treatment for infertility. Even in 1995, the steps involved with each of these processes are confusing and unclear for couples needing assistance with the reproductive process. This has led to a great deal of wasted time, money, energy, and pain for thousands of North American couples, particularly in the United States, where most procedures for infertility treatment are not covered by health insurance.

One area in need of improvement is the lack of *self-education* regarding fertility awareness and reproduction. Many couples do not understand what their "homework assignments" *really* are when it comes to preconception planning. In addition to timing intercourse to coincide with ovulation, a couple needs to screen out several conditions that may interfere with a pregnancy or with initial conception. In fact, many of the same problems that threaten a pregnancy affect a couple's fertility.

Another area that needs to be addressed is choosing an appropriate "fertility doctor," which is the subject of chapter 1. Because, in some countries other than the U.S., fertility is not a specialty that requires specific board-certification, the number of doctors and scientists who consider themselves "fertility specialists" is staggering. Knowing who the right specialist is and *when* to seek out that specialist is often the biggest obstacle for couples. And, once a couple finds the appropriate specialist, knowing how to "use" the specialist properly is another gray area. For example, although male and female fertility problems are evenly split, it is often the woman who becomes the fertility "contractor" for a couple, going alone for initial fertility counseling and even subjecting herself to a full, invasive fertility "workup" (discussed in chapter 5) without her partner's participation. As clearly stated in this book's first chapter, it takes two to make a baby—even if it's in a petrie dish! Understanding how to utilize a fertility specialist as a *united couple* is essential for successful diagnosis and treatment of fertility problems.

Knowing when to walk away is a crucial factor in fertility treatment. This is a decision that, believe it or not, really *begins* the treatment process instead of ending it. Setting up realistic goals and limits before fertility treatment begins is the key to success. In fact, this book attempts to re-define "success" when it comes to this issue. A couple who has gone through three IVF (in vitro fertilization) attempts and has not conceived but chooses to stop treatment is just as "successful" as a couple who "hits the jackpot" and conceives with the first IVF attempt. In both cases, the couples have gone beyond the call of duty to biologically parent a child. The fact that only one effort ends in a conception does not define "success"; it is the couple's *commitment* to the process that does. Both are successful in that they have dared to challenge their own biological limits. *No one can ask for more than that when it comes to fertility.* Sometimes, walking away from treatment takes more courage and self-sacrifice than staying in it.

This book also sheds light on how the infertility epidemic affects both men and women. For women, the fundamentals of family planning revolve around basic fertility awareness. However, because of the availability of hormonal contraception and the widespread use of condoms and other barrier methods, the ability to *read* one's menstrual cycles accurately and time intercourse to either prevent or create a pregnancy has become a lost art. In our society, healthy discomforts of a normal menstrual cycle are often medicated. Women who suffer from normal premenstrual symptoms, such as bloating or premenstrual breast pain, may be put on medications that elimi-nate their symptoms and, in more extreme cases, halt or alter their cycles. Yet these classic pre-menstrual symptoms are important *clues* to the timing of the cycle. By masking these symptoms, we are *masking the cycle.* (See chapter 3 for more details.)

This trend in women's health care is contributing to decreased fertility awareness and creat-ing problems for women on both sides of the fertility battle. Because less women are using more natural methods of birth control, they are subjected to certain risks that come with various con-traceptives, such as IUDs (intrauterine devices). Women who *do* want to conceive may find that their natural, "un-induced" cycles are not as predictable or easy to read as they thought. In most cases, women need to be *taught* how to read their cycles. This takes time and energy and often re-sults in a long wait for conception.

For both males and females, past sexual behavior and contraceptive history is also a huge factor in infertility. For example, when it comes to female-related infertility, 20% is due to an ir-regular ovulation cycle, accompanied by poor cervical mucus (see chapters 3 and 5). There are replacement hormones and/or drugs available that can induce ovulation (see chapter 7). In some geographic centers, as much as 80% of female infertility is due to scarring of the tubes from PID (pelvic inflammatory disease) caused by gonorrhea, chlamydia, and IUDs; and from endometrio-sis. Some of this scarring can be reversed through microsurgical techniques now available (dis-cussed in chapter 6). In essence, at least 50% of all female infertility can be prevented through safe sex.

Of course, STDs (sexually transmitted diseases) can also render males sterile because many infections interfere with semen production. Infections of the prostate and urinary tract (causing prostitis or urethritis) can cause male infertility. If left untreated, these infections not only will be passed on to his female partner, but also could cause future health problems for the male, including prostate trouble.

Finally, it's important to address the rather broad term of *infertility*. Technically, it means either conception is being *delayed* for some reason, or a pregnancy cannot be *sustained* (see chapter 9). However, people tend to confuse the word *infertility* with *sterility*. There is a *huge* difference between the two terms; infertility refers to a transient, or temporary state, whereas sterility denotes a more permanent state, although this state can often be reversed.

A couple is considered infertile if a pregnancy doesn't occur after one year of unprotected intercourse. Under ideal conditions, only 42% of a normal fertile woman's cycles will result in a full-term pregnancy from a fertile partner. *Currently, about one in seven couples will not conceive after one year of unprotected sex.* Ninety percent of the time, there is a physical cause behind this delayed conception: 35% of the time, the cause involves the man; 35% of the time, the cause involves the woman; 20% of the time the cause involves both partners; for the remaining 10% of time, no cause can be found.

Roughly 20% of North American couples are plagued by infertility. It's believed that about 3.5 million couples in North America are definitely sterile; about 3 million are considered subfertile, meaning not as fertile as the average couple, but *not* sterile, while about 1.5 million couples can expect a long wait before conception.

When a couple is sterile, it means there is a *permanent* physical phenomenon at work that is preventing pregnancy. Unless corrected through surgery, or other therapies, the problem *will* persist. (Correcting permanent problems is discussed in chapter 6.) Sometimes the problem is not correctable. In these cases, couples can consider options to pregnancy or assisted conception techniques. Of course, some men or women deliberately seek out permanent methods of contraception that *will* render them sterile. This book assumes that you have no history of either a vasectomy or tubal ligation procedure.

Infertility is caused by a combination of factors that, when examined individually, are not obstacles to conception. For example, virtually every woman is working, subjected to stress that was not present 30 years ago. As a result, women are more exhausted and emotionally drained than their mothers were at their age, and their partners are more exhausted and emotionally drained than their fathers were at their age. Furthermore, couples are planning first pregnancies at a much older age than their parents did. These factors are not causes of infertility but may certainly contribute to delayed fertility or problem pregnancies for many women.

I've designed this book as a step-by-step source to learning more about your fertility. It begins with the assumption that you're fertile until proven otherwise, and reveals the proper steps to take in conception planning and finding the appropriate specialists to guide you (see chapter 1). Chapter 2 outlines lifestyle habits that may be interfering with conception. In chapter 3 you'll learn how to read your ovulation cycle correctly, and how to time intercourse to coincide with the cycle. Chapters 4 and 5 cover the fertility investigation in detail, outlining what's involved in both the male workup (chapter 4) and the female workup (chapter 5). Chapter 6 is devoted to all the possible explanations for infertility, based on results of various tests discussed in chapters 4 and 5, and describes current treatments. In chapter 7 the focus is on fertility drugs, including the side effects and effectiveness of each drug, how the drug is administered, and costs and dosages in various scenarios. Chapter 8 discusses more elaborate fertility treatments, such as assisted reproductive technologies, and covers everything you need to know about the latest procedures and their success rates. Pregnancy loss—a risk every fertility patient takes—is the subject of chapter 9. Chapter 10 is devoted to alternatives: refusal of treatment, adoption, and childfree living.

For most of you, there is a logical explanation behind your infertility that is easily correctable. Whether your fertility journey ends in an alternative lifestyle, conception, miscarriage, or birth, I hope this book will help you with the most important issue of all: *your* life.

Who is a Fertility Doctor, and When Do You Need One?

If you've never had a child, you're probably curious about the state of your reproductive organs. That's only natural in light of the fact that we are in the midst of an infertility epidemic. The funny thing about this infertility epidemic, though, is that we really can't prove that it exists. Interpreting the statistics regarding fertility rates (production of children) and fecundity rates (the capacity to reproduce) can be tricky. For example, if we simply look at birthrate statistics, there's no doubt that they've declined since the late 1950s and early 1960s. But that's because there has been a major upheaval in the size of families and the nature of "family." Couples are marrying later in life, fewer people are marrying, fewer married women are having children, women are having fewer children, and more first pregnancies are occurring in women over 35—which, not so long ago, used to be the "cutoff" date for childbearing.

Another problem with comparing past and present birthrates is that we really haven't had a major war lately, which may have brought about the same furious wave of lovemaking and conceptions as the post–World War II baby boom did. In other words, social and political conditions have a huge effect on fertility statistics.

Beginning around the mid-1980s, we began to experience a second-wave baby boom that brought about a significant rise in fertility rates—a rise not seen since the 1950s. Obviously the children of the first baby boom had grown up and were having children themselves. But they were having *fewer* children than were the couples of the 1950s and early 1960s, and *fewer* of these first-wave boomers were even having children in the first place. There are so many first-wave boomers that *any* reproductive activity on their part profoundly affected the almost stagnant birthrate of the time. We also have no way of knowing how many of the newborns included in this second wave were conceived through assisted conception techniques, the aid of fertility drugs, spontaneous lovemaking, or carefully planned lovemaking. Furthermore, how many of these births were to teenage mothers? How many births were *wanted*? Remember, in today's social trends, more teenagers are sexually active, resulting in more teenage pregnancies and unplanned births.

What can we prove about fertility by examining the rate of "nonbirths?" For example, in the late 1980s, a study in Sweden by Princeton University and Lunds University revealed that the rate of childless white women was no higher in 1981 than it was in 1941. (Remember, the attack on Pearl Harbor didn't happen until December. In the United States, there were plenty of white men around until about January 1942.) The same study revealed that the rate of childless non-white women over the age of 30 has dropped since the 1950s. Again, the social trends of the times greatly affect this statistic. The *real* translation: Less white women got pregnant during the Great Depression (which really wasn't over in the United States until 1941, when the Americans entered the war). And since the 1950s, more nonwhite women have joined the poverty line, gotten pregnant as teenagers, or gotten pregnant as a way to get more money through government assistance. (Single mothers with no higher education in North America can make more money on welfare with two or more children than they can *working* to support *one* child!) So much for *that* study.

As for fecundity, here's what the statisticians have to say: If you compare women of the same age from the 1960s and the 1980s, their capacity to reproduce remains at exactly the same rate. Because women in the 1980s are choosing to have children at an older age, however, the overall infertility rate has risen. A 19-year-old woman today is just as fertile as a 19-year-old woman in 1960; a 40-year-old woman today is just as fertile (and probably in better shape) as a 40-year-old woman in 1960. But more 40-year-olds in the 1980s (and even more in 1995) desire pregnancy than did the 40-year-olds of 1960, and more 40-year-olds in the 1980s and today desire pregnancy than do the 19-year-olds of today. Therefore, more women are having difficulty conceiving today than in the 1960s.

There's another wrinkle we need to add to the fecundity statistic: More 19-year-old men *and* women were having unprotected sex with multiple partners in the 1970s and 1980s than they were in the 1950s and 1960s. As as result, more people in their 30s and 40s today have sexually transmitted diseases (STDs), which can or did wreak havoc on their fecundity.

What do all these confusing statistics have to do with your own fertility? Probably nothing. In the same way that one is assumed innocent until proven guilty, one is assumed to be fertile until proven otherwise. That means that before you can start investigating why you may not be able to conceive, you must have solid, concrete proof to support your suspicions of infertility in the *first* place. (Again, infertility, as stressed in this book's introduction, can mean anything from delayed conception to temporary or permanent barriers to conception.) In other words, you shouldn't graduate to a "fertility doctor" until you do the groundwork. The first part of this chapter explains what this groundwork really involves when it comes to conception—because unless you've done *yours*, a fertility doctor cannot do *his* or *hers*.

The second part of this chapter focuses on who the appropriate fertility specialist is (which depends on who has the problem), what the appropriate diagnostic steps are, and when you need to see various specialists in the conception planning process. Finally, we discuss how to "use" a fertility specialist, which is a must if our fertility workups are to be successful.

The Groundwork

I liken the conception process to yardwork. There are several things you need to weed out before your yard is pronounced "healthy." Similarly, there are several physical problems *you* need to weed out before you can really begin "trying." Unless you're prepared to do this yardwork, a proper fertility workup cannot be done.

Preconception Weeding

Although many couples think the first step in conception planning is to take a crash course in menstrual cycle mechanics (discussed further below and in chapter 3), this actually a a *later* step. The absolute first step in conception planning is pulling out the weeds that may interfere with or make you question conception. In short, *pull the weeds before you conceive!*

To do the necessary weeding, you'll need a "weed doctor." *Who* is this person? It depends where you live. Anywhere in Canada, or in smaller communities in the United States that are far from large medical centers, a primary care physician can do the "weeding." In larger urban centers in the United States, the task of weeding is best performed by either a genetic counselor (who any primary care physician can refer you to) or a gynecologist. A *primary care physician* can be an internist, general practitioner, or family practitioner.

You and your partner should see the weed doctor together. That way, one doctor will be managing all of the necessary screenings and histories for both of you. At all times, if a woman is seeing a gynecologist whom she's comfortable with, the gynecologist may do the "weeding" for both partners as well. It is a *mistake* to seek out *any* kind of fertility specialist until this weeding process is completed.

Weeding consists of being screened for a number of problems at the outset of your conception journey rather than the middle or at the end. The time you take to be screened now could save you months or years of frustration. If a problem is discovered now, you'll have more time to correct it. If no problem is found and if you don't conceive within a reasonable amount of time, you'll be able to cross a number of possible problems off the list. You can then get to the bottom of your conception delay much sooner. Finally, if you do get pregnant soon after the weeding, you'll have taken every precaution to prevent or prepare for a high-risk pregnancy.

Depending on the results of the screenings, however, one or both of you may be *referred* to a specialist. In the case of a primary care doctor, his or her role is to manage your *overall* health. In other words, primary care doctors specialize in being *generalists*. When the time comes, they will refer you to the appropriate specialist—be it a "fertility" specialist, a gynecologist, an obstetrician, or even a perinatalogist (specializing in high-risk pregnancies).

You probably will be screened for the following:

Several genetic disorders

Don't even *think* about having children until you've been checked for genetic disorders. You can be a carrier of a disorder even if you are not personally affected by it. Some examples of these disorders are Tay-Sachs disease (if you're Jewish or French Canadian); sickle cell anemia (if you're of Mediterranean or African descent); certain diseases linked to the X chromosome (in other words, diseases carried by the female and passed on to her male child, such as various forms of muscular dystrophy including leukodystrophies and hemophilia). When you present yourself to your doctor and tell him or her that you'd like to be screened for any possible genetic or chromosomal disorders, he or she will take it from there. Your race and family history will determine which diseases you need to be screened for. If you happen to be a carrier of a disease linked to the X chromosome, you'll need to go for genetic counseling and weigh the risks of even having a child, as well as prepare for various prenatal tests during a pregnancy. If you carry any genetic diseases that require *both* you and partner to be carriers before the genes can be passed on (such as Tay-Sachs), then your partner MUST be screened as well. If you're both carriers, you'll also need genetic counseling before you venture into the "trying" phase.

Rh incompatibility

Your blood type is either Rh positive (meaning you have an Rh factor in your blood, as 85% of us do) or Rh negative (meaning you don't have an Rh factor). Either is fine, *but* if the male partner is Rh positive and the female partner is Rh negative, the blood type of your offspring may not match *the mother's*. If not diagnosed, this can be a big problem during delivery or even in the event of a pregnancy loss or therapeutic abortion. However, once diagnosed, medications such as Rhogam can fix the problem.

German measles (rubella)

When you're planning a pregnancy, it's important to screen out rubella. In early pregnancy, this disease can damage the fetus. Most women (1 in 7) were vaccinated long ago for rubella but may not remember the vaccine. Women can be screened for a rubella *titer*, a test that detects whether antibodies to rubella are present in the bloodstream. If you have the antibodies, you're immune; if you don't, you'll need to consult with your doctor about the next step, which usually involves a vaccine.

Human immunodeficiency virus (HIV)

If you have reason to suspect that you've been exposed to HIV, you must take an HIV antibody test if you're planning pregnancy. Review the risk groups and risk factors with your doctor, or call your local AIDS hotline.

Chlamydia

If you have chlamydia, you'll need to make sure it is treated before you try to conceive. (Even so, 10% of the time, people who have chlamydia will test negative for it.) Chlamydia is one of the most common STDs in North America right now, and in the sexually active 18–30 crowd, as many as 50% *have chlamydia*. Chlamydia is particularly nasty because it is usually *asymptomatic* (meaning it has no symptoms). In one year, about 4.5 million women in North America will be infected with chlamydia, and 60% of them will not have any symptoms. But the disease can do a lot of damage and lead to *pelvic inflammatory disease* (PID), discussed in chapter 6, which is a primary cause of female infertility. Some experts estimate that chlamydia causes 50% of all pelvic infections and 25% of all tubal pregnancies (ectopic pregnancies) due to scarring and/or inflammation of the fallopian tubes. (Inflammation of the tubes is called *salpingitis*.) Chlamydia can also cause urethral infections in both men and women, and cervicitis (inflammation of the cervix) in women.

The screening is simple. Your doctor takes a culture swab of cervical mucus. It can be done in conjunction with a Pap test. Chlamydia is *extremely* easy to treat: Tetracycline will cure it. The drug usually prescribed is *doxycycline* (Vibramycin), which is a derivative of *tetracycline* (Tetracyn and many other brands). Two doxycycline capsules per day ten days will do the trick. Tetracycline, which is cheaper, must be taken four times a day, but many people forget to take that many pills; that's why doxycycline is better. If you're already pregnant or cannot be on tetracycline, you'll be given *erythromycin* (Eryc, PCE, Erythromid, and many others). Incidentally, as many as 10% of all pregnant women are found to have chlamydia, which can cause a host of problems during pregnancy and delivery.

Gonorrhea

Gonorrhea is another STD that's fairly common and does more damage to women than to men. If left untreated, gonorrhea can cause PID as well and subsequent female infertility. *It is believed that gonorrhea and chlamydia account for 80% of all PID.* However, gonorrhea is *less* common than chlamydia. If a woman is diagnosed with gonorrhea, she'll also be treated for chlamydia. The reasoning: "If she managed to catch gonorrhea, she's got an enormous chance of already having chlamydia. Better treat her for both just in case!" In fact, women can often be simultaneously infected with both chlamydia and gonorrhea if the partner is a carrier for both infections. After one sexual contact with an infected partner, women have a 30% chance of contracting gonorrhea and almost a 100% chance if they are on hormonal contraception. Like chlamydia, early-stage gonorrhea is asymptomatic about 80% of the time. Symptoms depend on where the gonococcal bacteria are "living."

During an annual pelvic exam, the doctor will check the cervix for any unusual discharge and often take a culture as a routine screening. Gonorrhea tests usually are 90% accurate if a culture test is done; if only a "gram stain" is performed, in which the discharge is smeared onto a slide and stained, the test is only 50% accurate for women, but very accurate for *men with symptoms*. In men, gonorrhea can lead to sterility as their bodies may develop sperm antibodies after they've been infected. When this happens, sperm motility is reduced, which affects male fertility.

The best thing to do if you suspect gonorrhea is to request two culture tests one week apart. If you *do* have gonorrhea, you will be either screened for chlamydia or simply treated for it. Gonorrhea is easily treated with antibiotics. One dose of *ceftriaxone* (Rocephin) and a follow-up prescription of doxycycline cures the probable chlamydia.

Mycoplasma

Mycoplasma (a.k.a. *Ureaplasma urealyticum*) is an asymptomatic bacterial infection that is more often than not, an STD. (In other words, virgins don't usually get mycoplasma!) Your doctor can detect mycoplasma by culturing cervical mucus during a routine Pap smear. It's important to be screened for mycoplasma prior to pregnancy because if left untreated, mycoplasma can travel to the endometrium, causing inflammation. This is known as *endometritis*—not to be confused with endometriosis. If you were pregnant with endometritis, the embryo may not implant in the uterus, and you would miscarry.

Herpes

Herpes is an STD caused by the herpes simplex virus. The virus enters the body through the skin and mucous membranes of the mouth and genitals and permanently sets up shop at the base of the spine.

There are two types of herpes: herpes simplex virus type I (HSV I), which is characterized by cold sores and fever blisters on the mouth and face, and herpes simplex virus type II (HSV II), the dreaded genital herpes. HSV I can be transmitted through kissing. You can also contract an HSV I and II "combo" if you have both oral sex and intercourse with an infected partner. Herpes *is* contagious whether the sores are active or not; it is most contagious when the sores are active, but has been found that most infection takes place when the sores are *inactive*. This is when herpes is known to be asymptomatic. When the sores are active they're visible and stand as a warning to the other partner "not to touch." Indeed the sores are so potent that touching them with the fingers and then touching the skin of a healthy person will transmit the virus. Even if there are no visible sores, the virus can still be transmitted.

The herpes sores are called vesicles, and they are painful, watery blisters that occur anywhere from 2–20 days after infection. Within a few days, the vesicles rupture, leaving behind shallow blisters that may ooze or bleed. After 3 or 4 days, scabs form and the vesicles fall off, healing by themselves without treatment.

There is no cure for herpes, but there are some antiviral medications (pills) that can help alleviate the pain. The initial outbreaks also take longer to heal, lasting about two to three weeks. Then, the virus will start to taper off, and you may go from monthly initial outbreaks to annual outbreaks. The usual pattern is nasty initial outbreaks, and milder recurrent episodes within 3–12 months after the first outbreak. Recurrences then become milder and far more sporadic, like once every two years and so on. Generally, factors such as stress, poor diet, caffeine, and hormonal elements (menstruation, oral contraceptives, and so on) trigger herpes outbreaks. The presence of other infections, such as vaginitis (inflammation of the vagina), genital warts, or yeast can also trigger a recurrence. Usually, there aren't any recurrences with HSV I. About 25% of people with HSV II may also never experience a recurrence.

Diagnosing herpes isn't difficult. When the sores are active, it's usually obvious. A blood test can detect whether you have herpes antibodies present. The problem with this test is that it can only tell you that you've contracted herpes at some point; it does not tell you when the initial infection occurred.

More than 30 million North Americans are currently infected with herpes, but only about 25% know they have it. Roughly 30% of the general population have been exposed to HSV II. If you've been exposed to herpes and are planning a pregnancy, ask your primary care physician for advice. The risk of passing on herpes to your spouse or partner years after an initial outbreak may be quite low if you don't suffer from recurrent herpes. Many women with herpes go on to have normal, healthy pregnancies and deliveries, but it's more important to rule out a herpes infection in the cervical area.

For more information on herpes and pregnancy, call the Herpes Resource Center hotline: (919) 361-8488.

Human papillomavirus (genital warts)

Genital warts are also STDs and are sometimes referred to as venereal warts. They are caused by the human papillomavirus (HPV). This virus is very similar to the one that causes skin warts, but there are more than twenty types of HPV floating around. Warts are painless and can appear on the vulva or the cervix or on a man's penis. Unless the warts are on the cervix, your doctor can usually spot them and treat them with a solution that will burn the wart off. HPV on the cervix can take the form of raised (condyloma) or flat lesions. Both types of lesions can be detected through a Pap smear. If left untreated, HPV can cause the cells on the lining of the cervix to change, which can lead to cervical cancer. HPV is currently *the* most common STD in North America. It is rampant in sexually active couples ages 18–35. HPV can be treated but never technically cured. Once the warts are removed, the virus generally doesn't cause problems, but it remains in your bloodstream forever. For women, follow-up Pap smears for the first couple of years after HPV diagnosis, and annual Pap smears after that, will help nip HPV in the bud should it decide to erupt again (which is an extremely rare event). When HPV is treated, however, you are in effect "cured." For both sexes, treatment can encompass cryosurgery or laser surgery, and for women, a sloughing cream can also be applied to the cervix.

Syphilis

Perhaps the most famous STD, syphilis was once a very serious, incurable disease that often resulted in "madness." Today it's easily treated with antibiotics. Syphilis is caused by a bacterium known as a *spirochete*. There are three stages of syphilis: primary, secondary, and tertiary (late-stage). It's transmitted through sexual or skin contact with someone who is already infected.

While syphilis does not cause infertility, when you're pregnant, you can transmit the disease to your unborn child, which is known as *congenital syphilis*. The number of congenital syphilis cases reported in 1988 was the highest since the early 1950s, and in New York City alone, the number had increased more than 500%! Untreated syphilis during pregnancy can lead to fetal bone and tooth deformities, fetal nerve damage, stillbirth, and fetal brain damage. All couples planning pregnancy should request a syphilis test. Syphilis spreads through open sores called *chancres* or rashes that pass through the mucous membrane lining the mouth, genitals, anus, or broken skin.

In the 1970s, syphilis was virtually eliminated as an STD because it had been aggressively treated in previous decades. In 1985, however, the incidence of syphilis skyrocketed in the United States and continues to rise.

Diagnosing syphilis is tricky. Known as the "great masquerader," syphilis symptoms imitate other symptoms and can be misdiagnosed. Syphilis is diagnosed through a blood test that checks for antibodies to spirochetes in the bloodstream. Two tests are involved; the first one screens for it, the second confirms it. Syphilis is a miserable, damaging disease that is *curable* with simple antibiotics, either penicillin or tetracycline. After you've been treated for syphilis at any stage, you'll need to have a follow-up test to make sure you've been cured.

Hepatitis B

Hepatitis B is a virus that causes inflammation of the liver. It's most common in people ages 15–39 and is a serious STD that is on the rise. It is transmitted through contaminated needles or blood, but it is also transmitted through mucus-sharing activities that involve saliva, semen, or vaginal fluid, which enter the bloodstream of an uninfected person. *Mothers can also pass on this virus to newborns during childbirth.*

It can take up to 180 days after infection for any hepatitis symptoms to develop. Most people who get hepatitis B remain well, have no symptoms, and completely recover. Even if you're asymptomatic, the virus can cause damage to the liver, which can lead to serious illness and even death. Those who *do* get sick generally experience flulike symptoms, jaundice, dark urine and light stools. Generally you will recover from hepatitis, but if you're unlucky the illness can overwhelm you for several months. Some people will always carry the hepatitis B virus and thus remain infectious.

There is no cure for hepatitis B, but there is a vaccine! Safe sex is *not* considered adequate protection from hepatitis B; only a hepatitis B vaccine will protect you. Like HIV, hepatitis B can flourish in an anal sex "environment" and among drug users. However, tattooing and ear piercing are also common routes of infection. Those at highest risk for hepatitis B are intravenous drug users, gay men, health care workers, and prostitutes.

The vaccine is given by injection in three doses over a six-month time period. The second shot is given one month after the first shot; the third shot is given five months after the second. Other than a sore arm for a day or two, side effects from the vaccine are rare. If you do suffer from any side effects, you'll experience general feelings of "unwellness," fatigue, and so on. Contact the physician or clinic that administered the vaccine.

Vaginal infections: Attention, Ladies

All vaginal infections should be treated prior to the "trying" phase, or else you will *not* be able to observe the cervical mucus accurately, nor will sexual intercourse be comfortable.

The most common vaginal infection is caused by the overgrowth of vaginal yeast known as *candidiasis*. This is *not* an STD. *Trichomoniasis* and *bacterial vaginosis* are also common, and can be passed on to a male partner during intercourse. All three infections are characterized by unusual, odorous vaginal discharge; cottage cheese–like discharge, coupled with the smell of baking bread, is often a classic symptom of a yeast infection.

Trichomoniasis is diagnosed by swabbing the vaginal discharge and examining it under the microscope. But "trich" can also cause urinary tract infections and can be passed back and forth between partners. Like both chlamydia and gonorrhea, if left untreated, trich can hitchhike up the fallopian tubes and cause Pelvic Inflammatory Disease and eventual infertility. Sixty percent of women with trich are cured with an antifungal medication called *clotrimazole* (Canestan). Women taking medication for "trich" must make sure that their partners are treated as well.

For bacterial vaginosis, the treatment for both partners is with a drug known as *metronidazole*. (Pregnant women are given a different drug in a suppository form.) The male partner must wear a condom until cured.

Yeast and trich aren't dangerous to a developing fetus per se, but could aggravate natural discomforts of pregnancy considerably. Bacterial vaginosis, however, can complicate a pregnancy if untreated and can trigger premature labor.

Group B Streptococcal Disease

In women, Group B streptococcus is a bacteria that normally lives in the vagina or rectum, along with a whole batch of other bacteria. Group B is a problem because it causes strep throat, scarlet fever, and some pneumonias. About 30% of all women have Group B strep, but they don't necessarily have any kind of infection. Normally, this doesn't pose any problems to your health, but when you're pregnant it can cause serious problems either during pregnancy or after childbirth. If you have a history of STDs, have given birth to children infected with Group B, or have a history of premature labor, you're more likely to be a Group B carrier. To date, routine screening for Group B strep isn't done due to a number of obstacles that have to do with practicality and feasibility. However, all women planning pregnancy should discuss with their physician whether they need to be screened for Group B strep given their individual risk profile.

Full physical

Both partners should have a full physical when planning pregnancy to make sure that their blood pressure, iron levels (for women), blood sugar, urine, cholesterol levels, heart rates, and so forth are all normal. The purpose is to establish that both partners are healthy and presumed fertile unless a problem is found. At this point, they should also discuss nutritional issues that may increase fertility, eliminating certain foods, tobacco, or alcohol while stockpiling on others. Make sure you bring along your family and personal medical history so your doctor can keep an eye on anything unusual. (Family/personal history charts are discussed further below.)

Autoimmune disorders

Autoimmune means "self-attacking." Most autoimmune disorders are hereditary but can affect a couple's fertility if left untreated. Common autoimmune diseases include diabetes, thyroid disease, lupus, and rheumatoid arthritis. The symptoms of these diseases may interfere temporarily with fertility until the diseases are brought under control through medication. For example, thyroid disease can interfere with regular ovulation and can reduce sperm count. A classic symptom of diabetes in women is chronic vaginal yeast infections, which will interfere with cervical mucus observation. Know your family history as well as the early warning signs of these illnesses so you can be screened for them.

History 101

When it comes to laying the groundwork, History 101 is a prerequisite, not an option! Both you and your partner will need to write a complete family and personal medical history that can be given to your "weed doctor." Should you need to see a fertility specialist later on, this history will help speed up the fertility treatment process tremendously. Here are the questions you'll need to address:

1. *Have there been previous pregnancies and/or abortions?* Has *he* impregnated someone in the past (with or without her knowledge)? Has *she* been pregnant (with or without his knowledge)? For example, many abortions performed in the 1970s were not performed

under the most sanitary conditions. Yet even when performed by experienced abortionists, scarring may have resulted that could be affecting your fertility now. Previous miscarriages and any subsequent D & Cs (*dilatation and curettage*, in which the the uterine lining is scraped out) may have also resulted in scarring. If you're a male who has impregnated another woman in the past, it's highly unlikely that you're infertile today unless you are taking certain medications known to reduce fertility or you have been exposed to certain toxins.

    And finally, any history of ectopic pregnancy may have resulted in tubal damage or even the removal of one or both tubes. This information is crucial to disclose!

2. *Do either of you have a history of pelvic surgeries or therapies?* Women who have had pelvic surgery or therapy of any kind (D & Cs, removal of ovarian cysts, treatment for cervical dysplasia, or laparoscopy procedures) need to disclose this information. Men who have had surgery in or around their genital area (for instance, removal of cysts around the testes) need to disclose this information too. Again, scarring from previous surgeries or procedures may be affecting your fertility now.

3. *Do you have a history of pelvic infection or pelvic pain?* Any woman who suffers from *chronic* pelvic pain (this does *not* mean menstrual cramps) may be suffering from pelvic inflammatory disease (PID). Any woman suffering from: menstrual cramps painful enough to keep her from participating in pleasurable activities, pelvic pain, constipation, or other pelvic discomforts during menstruation may have endometriosis. Both PID and endometriosis can affect your pelvic organs and in some cases can interfere with ovarian function. You MUST report these symptoms if you have them.

4. *Do either of you have a history of cancer therapy?* Anticancer drugs and chemotherapy *can* affect future fertility for both men and women. Both testicular and ovarian function can be permanently affected. Some common cancers in younger adults that require chemotherapy treatments include Hodgkin's disease, leukemia, breast cancer, testicular cancer (relevant when one testicle remains), and non-Hodgkin's lymphoma. Of course, there are many other kinds of cancers for which either of you may have received chemotherapy treatments. External radiation therapy will not affect your fertility unless the radiation beam was directed at the ovaries or testicles.

5. *What is your hormonal contraceptive history?* Were you ever on combination oral contraceptives or the mini-pill? Norplant? Depo-Provera? In each case, how many years were you on hormonal contraception? Have your menstrual cycles returned to normal? (See chapter 3 for more details on the menstrual cycle and hormonal contraceptives.)

Women with a long history of hormonal contraception may have a more difficult time getting pregnant. This has more to do with waiting for the return of normal menstrual cycles than any permanent infertility.

6. *What is your history of hormonal therapy?* Were you prescribed estrogen or progesterone for any reason? Were you ever on *Danazol* (a male hormone derivative that shuts down ovarian function—sometimes used to treat endometriosis)? Were you taking hormonal therapy as part of any cancer treatment (such as *tamoxifen*)? Hormonal therapy will most definitely interfere with normal ovulation, but this interference is temporary. Once you go off the medication, your menstrual cycle should resume, but you may need to stay on hormonal therapy to treat a more serious condition. Discuss your options with the doctor who is managing your therapy.

7. *What is your contraceptive history in general?* Have you ever used an IUD? What barrier methods have you used? IUDs are particularly suspicious because they can trigger bacterial infections that lead to PID (discussed in detail in chapter 6). Your condom history is also important because this will give your doctor an idea of your risk factor for exposure to STDs. Attention, men: Your condom history is important as well.

8. *Assuming neither of you have an STD today, have either of you ever been treated for an STD in the past?* This is more of a concern for women than for men. Even if a woman was already been treated for chlamydia or gonorrhea, she may *still* have suffered tubal damage as a result. That's why it's crucial that you're both screened for STDs! Screening today will also ensure that past treatments worked.

9. *Do either of you suffer from chronic bladder or urinary tract infections?* This spells I-N-F-E-C-T-I-O-N. Men who have cloudy urine or experience a burning sensation when they urinate may have *nongonococcal urethritis* (NGU) (inflammation of the urethra that is *not* caused by gonorrhea, a.k.a. nonspecific urethritis). When a man has NGU, he almost *always* has chlamydia, which can be passed on to his partner. She in turn may not show any symptoms, creating an STD merry-go-round of nightmarish proportions.

   On the other hand, women who suffer from symptoms of UTIs (urinary tract infections) may have cystitis (a bladder infection, which could affect the kidneys if left untreated), a vaginal infection, or an STD. Be on the lookout for painful urination, frequent urination, and either or both symptoms in conjunction with a sluggish or almost nonexistent urine stream and fever.

10. *Do either of you have a family history of only children? Did either mother have a late pregnancy or a history of troubled pregnancies?* The answers to these questions may mean nothing, or

they may be clues to a family history of pregnancy or fertility *complications*. For example, diseases such as endometriosis (discussed in chapter 6) are hereditary, but women who suffer from endometriosis often have no symptoms. Some problems that cause male infertility may be hereditary, and so on. The bottom line is that knowing your parents' fertility history will help your doctor probe further and ask more direct questions, which may yield more definite answers for you!

11. *Are either of you DES children?* Anyone born in the United States between 1941 and 1971 (perhaps even a little beyond that) may be a DES daughter or DES son. During this period, five million pregnant women took the drug *DES* (*diethylstilbestrol*, a synthetic estrogen) to prevent miscarriage. Any daughter born to a mother who took DES runs a higher than normal risk for reproductive organ abnormalities (such as twisted fallopian tubes), cervical and vaginal cell changes, and cancer. All this can spell trouble when she tries to conceive. Men who are DES sons may also have anatomical abnormalities when it comes to their reproductive organs, although DES sons are not as commonly affected as are daughters.

    DES was administered under a host of different labels. If you can, find out the name of the drugs your mother took during her pregnancy and contact DES Action at (510) 465-4011. Ask them to check if any of the drugs you discovered match the drugs on their list. DES Action has a nationwide referral service of doctors who specialize in the treatment of DES-exposed women and men.

12. *Do either of you suffer from a chronic disease/condition such as diabetes, lupus, rheumatoid arthritis, thyroid disease, multiple sclerosis, asthma, ulcers, and so on?* Depending on your age and condition, pregnancy may not be recommended to begin with, or your condition may be affecting your fertility.

13. *Are either of you taking medications to control a chronic medical or psychiatric condition?* Many medications can interfere with fertility for both men and women, so you need to disclose *all* of this information to your primary care doctor. Certain antidepressants, any medications that contain steroids (used to control asthma, for example), and certain ulcer medications are classic examples.

14. *Have either of you been exposed to environmental toxins?* Exposure to radiation (also used in cancer therapy), toxic chemicals such as lead, pesticides, insecticides, polystyrene, xylene, benzene, mercury, Agent Orange, anesthetic gases, PCBs, or solvents can cause both temporary or, in extreme cases, permanent damage to your reproductive organs. (Are either of you Gulf War veterans?) Often just getting away from a toxic environ-

ment can restore fertility. This is discussed further in chapter 2.

15. *What are your lifestyle and nutritional habits and vices?* This is something you *really* need to explore and is the subject of chapter 2. As amazing as it may seem, cutting out certain foods and chemicals and changing habits can result in conception after months of delays.

A good primary care physician will most likely ask you these questions anyway, but addressing these issues yourselves beforehand will help you form a conception *partnership*. In addition, clearly reviewing your medical histories is an excellent way to prepare you for parenthood. Parents are the "health care contractors" for their children. Knowing your own histories will help you prepare or comfort your offspring should a future health problem arise.

When Do We Chart the Menstrual Cycle?

This is an excellent question, one to which many couples don't know the answer. At this point, you shouldn't be *trying* to conceive until you've done the weeding.

Even if your menstrual cycles *are* charted (see chapter 3) and are so regular that you can set your watch by them, *unless you've done your weeding and history lesson above, this will mean nothing and can waste months of time!* Fertility problems revolve around *structural* problems (his or hers) and *hormonal* problems (his or hers). Menstrual cycle abnormalities will identify female hormonal problems only—*which account for just a small portion of fertility problems in general*. Today, roughly 80% of all female infertility is due to structural damage to the fallopian tubes from PID. And, women with PID can have perfectly normal menstrual cycles. So, while understanding both the female and male hormonal cycles is crucial to conception (the female cycle is discussed in chapter 3; the male cycle is discussed in chapter 4), it is *not* the first step in conception *planning*.

If your screenings all came back negative (normal), then the next step is to read chapters 2 and 3. You're looking at about a year's worth of "trying" before you should even suspect there's a fertility problem.

If your screenings revealed a garden-variety weed of some sort (an STD or a suspected PID), you'll need to "treat and repeat." Treat the STD, go off the drugs that are making you infertile, and go for diagnostic tests to confirm the problem. You may need certain treatment or need to repeat certain tests before you complete your screening process. Then read chapters 2 and 3 and begin your "trying" phase.

The next section of this chapter may either be "in order" or "out of order" depending on how your screening process goes. Essentially, the "Groundwork" = Weeding + 1 Year of Trying (based on information in Chapters 2 and 3).

When the year is up and there's still no baby, both of you and your weed doctor may graduate to what's called a workup (discussed in chapters 4 and 5). The workup is a special series of tests that pinpoint hormonal, structural, or immunological problems that may be interfering with conception. Men and women require *different* workups. To avoid wasting time and money, *both* the male and female workups begin with a semen analysis—the easiest, cheapest, and least invasive test of all. Whoever is managing your preconception screening should manage the semen analysis. The results of the semen analysis will determine the next steps.

The "Fertility Doctor"

In 1995, no area has caused more confusion or lawsuits than fertility treatment. This is because there is no such thing as a fertility or infertility specialist per se—*yet*. In other words, a graduating M.D. cannot become a "board-certified fertility specialist" in the way that he or she can become a board-certified gynecologist or pediatrician. To date, no postgraduate board certification course exists for this purpose.

This, understandably, creates enormous problems for the fertility consumer. Essentially, any M.D or even Ph.D. can say that she or he is a fertility specialist, but this does not mean that he or she is *qualified* to treat a fertility problem.

The answer to "who is a fertility specialist?" is rather complicated. The doctor that manages your infertility workup will vary depending on who has the problem. Male infertility specialists are either *andrologists* (M.D.'s or Ph.D. scientists specializing in male fertility and in assisted reproductive technology) or *urologists* (doctors who specialize in male and female urinary tract problems but are particularly knowledgeable about penis and testicle "design"). Many urologists are also andrologists.

As I stress repeatedly throughout this book, both the male and the female workup begin with a semen analysis. If your partner has an abnormal semen analysis, he'll be sent for a "male workup," (discussed in chapter 4). If the semen analysis is normal, you'll then go on as a couple to a gynecologist who specializes in *reproductive endocrinology*. This person is qualified to manage the "female workup" (discussed in chapter 5).

If you and your partner decide to undergo assisted reproductive technology (see chapter 8), the following combination of specialists is appropriate: a gynecologist who subspecializes in reproductive endocrinology; a urologist (for male infertility) who subspecializes in andrology; an *em-*

bryologist (a Ph.D. scientist specializing in embryo transfers—this person should never manage the treatment, however).

A *radiologist* (a doctor specializing in imaging tests) can be called in as a consultant by your specialist, but you will rarely have occasion to meet him/her.

How to Find a Good Fertility Specialist

Never, I repeat, *never* go to a fertility specialist because he or she has been recommended by a friend. Picking the right fertility specialist greatly depends on who has the problem and what kind of treatment route you've decided to take. In the same way that real estate agents always sell you on "location, location, location," finding a good, *appropriate* fertility specialist depends on "referral, referral, referral." You *first* need a good primary care physician who can refer you to the appropriate specialist. This requires some medical diagnostic training—something that your friend's neighbor's sister *doesn't* have!

If you don't have a good primary physician but *do* have a good gynecologist, the gynecologist can serve as your "weed doctor" (as mentioned earlier) and can refer you to the appropriate specialist when the time comes. If this gynecologist subspecializes in reproductive endocrinology, then he of she can manage the female workup if need be.

You can also phone one of the infertility/fertility organizations listed at the back of this book and ask for a list of qualified reproductive endocrinologists, andrologists, urologists, and so on. Other ways of making short lists of potential specialists involve contacting former infertility patients from a patient support group, or contacting a specific hospital directly. Generally, seeking out a fertility specialist on your own should should be done only if you're unhappy with the referral from your "weed doctor" and if you already know *who* needs the workup. Otherwise, you could be wasting time and money.

This leads to an obvious question: How do you find that weed doctor to begin with? Two ways: "friends, friends, friends" or "referral, referral, referral." Ask someone whose opinion you value. Who do *they* see? Who does their *spouse* see? Or, if you have an allergist, podiatrist, or pulmonary specialist whom you really like, who do *they* recommend as a primary care doctor? Who is *their* doctor, or their *spouse's* doctor? You get the idea. You can also call the American Medical Association or, in Canada, the College of Physicians and Surgeons (the provincial branches) for lists of primary care physicians in your area. *NOTE: If you live away from a major medical center or urban area, you may need to travel to a center for your care. Infertility specialists are few and far between since this is a relatively new area of specialty.*

Going for a Test Drive

The results from your semen analyses (you need at least two) are back. You're now proceeding with either a male or female workup. Whether you're seeing an andrologist, reproductive endocrinologist, gynecologist, or urologist, here are the questions you need to ask at your first appointment as a way of "test driving" your specialist:

1. *Are you board-certified?* This means that he or she has completed a residency training program that has met with the standards set by the American board of that particular field (obstetrics and gynecology, endocrinology, urology, and so on). For example, there's a 1 in 2.5 chance that any gynecologist you see is not board-certified.

2. *What are your subspecialties?* Does your gynecologist "do" reproductive endocrinology? Does your urologist "do" andrology? Does your andrologist "do" urology?

3. *Who will manage the pregnancy if conception is achieved? (If you're seeing a gynecologist, does he or she do obstetrics?)* Because you're planning to get pregnant, you should have an obstetrician waiting in the wings. Also, if your treatment is successful, you *will* have a high-risk pregnancy and must be under the care of an obstetrician. A midwife or primary care doctor won't do!

4. *What kind of hospital privileges do you have?* Full operating privileges are best.

5. *Do you share copies of medical records and test results with your patients at their request?* If he or she won't, that's a bad sign.

6. *Are you available for occasional phone calls?* Find out if the doctor is accessible, or if you have to make an appointment just ask a question.

7. (If the specialist is male, and you're undergoing a female workup) *Is a female assistant present in the room when you perform a pelvic exam or administer treatment/testing in the pelvic area? If not, do you object if I bring along a friend or my spouse?* If the male doctor performs "solo pelvics," it's not only a bad sign, but it's illegal in most places. (Sorry, guys, there are no laws in place that call for a male nurse in the room while a female urologist examines your genitals. You may ask to bring your spouse, however. There are no laws covering same-sex doctor-patient exams either.)

8. *How much of your practice revolves around infertility treatment?* Does the urologist specialize in treating cystitis only but *dabbles* in male fertility? Does the reproductive endocrinologist have a waiting room filled with menopausal women and only *occasionally* handles the odd fertility workup? You'll want someone who focuses a good portion of his or her practice on fertility treatment.

9. *What are the costs involved?* Once you factor in the costs of both diagnostic procedures and treatments, you could be looking at a hefty price tag. You MUST get a rough estimate up front so you can make the necessary insurance arrangements for coverage. (In Canada, many procedures and therapies involving infertility are not covered by provincial health insurance. Find out what's covered before making your decisions.)

10. *How experienced are you in monitoring and administering fertility drugs?* Because these drugs are extrememly potent, you'll want a doctor who knows what he or she is doing when it comes to dosage monitoring, dosage adjusting, and side-effects. (See chapter 7 for more details.)

11. *Who will perform microsurgery?* If your fertility is being caused by a structual problem, such as blocked tubes in women, scrotal varicose veins in men, or reversal of vasectomy procedures, who will actually be *doing* the surgery? You may ask to meet with the surgeon at some point, too.

12. *What other services do you offer to patients?* Can you join a support group? Are counselors available? Are there videos or other reference materials? The more information you can sink your teeth into, the better.

13. *What percentage of live births have resulted from your treatments?* Be careful with the term *success rates* because many doctors or clinics won't distinguish pregnancies from actual births. Also, keep in mind that when a pregnancy is established, the rate of miscarriage is far higher under many of these specialized treatments than it is under standard treatment.

14. *What percentage of multiple pregnancies have resulted from your treatments?* This time, it's helpful to know how many past patients carried multiple fetuses. Multiple births are higher risk pregnancies and carry lower gestation periods. This is an important piece of data if you can get it. Ask, again, how many *live* multiple births resulted.

How to Use Your Fertility Specialist

The first rule in fertility treatment is: *Do it together.* If you're not seeing the doctor as a couple *united,* than you're already off to a bad start. As I discuss throughout this book, your fertility workup and treatment route is not just about one person, but two—*three* if the treatment is successful. Although a common scenario is for the woman to act as the couple's "fertility contractor" and visit the specialist alone, the only time a woman should go through fertility workups and treatment alone *is if she's single*. Otherwise, it takes two to make a baby, even if it's in a petri dish!

The second rule is: *100% disclosure*. Naturally, as fertility patients, *you* have to be responsible for making sure your doctor is acting in your best interests. To do this, you have to assert your rights and act responsibly. For example, if either of you keep information from each other or the doctor (such as previous abortions, previous paternity, colorful sexual histories, previous STDs), you can't expect your doctor to make an accurate diagnosis. Similarly, if you don't ask questions when you don't understand something, you can't expect your doctor to read your mind and explain things more clearly. Disclosure also comes into play later on, with symptoms or side effects to various drugs or treatments. Report all side effects, no matter how insignificant.

Finally, the third rule about fertility treatment is: *No one is God*. Only God (or a reasonable facsimile thereof) knows and controls the outcome of your fertility treatment. Your doctor isn't God, nor should he or she try to act like it; your partner isn't God, and you're not God. The only role your doctor plays is that of a "technician to the gods," who facilitates reproduction.

Keeping all of these points in mind, here's an example of how easily a fertility investigation can become a botched job, wasting everyone's time—something you don't have too much of when you're trying to get pregnant.

The Wrong Way to Use a Fertility Doctor

John and Jane, both in their early thirties, have been married for three years. Prior to their marriage, both had been sexually active since their teens. John's contraceptive history consisted of asking one question of his lovers: "Are you on the Pill?" By the time AIDS became an issue for him (circa 1990), he and Jane were already in a monogamous relationship.

Jane had been using oral contraceptives since her senior year in high school. After talking it over with John, she went off her contraceptives on her wedding night. Having tried unsuccessfully to get pregnant for the past two years, Jane decides to see her gynecologist. She goes alone, while John stays home. As it turns out, Jane's gynecologist, while board-certified, does *not* subspecialize in reproductive endocrinology, nor does he practice obstetrics. You might say that he's basically a "Pap and fibroid" man.

During her appointment, Jane's gynecologist asks her if she's had any preconception counselling. He's referring, of course, to all of the screenings and "weedings" outlined earlier in this chapter. Jane is embarrassed to admit that she doesn't *understand* what he means by this phrase, so she just says yes. The gynecologist then asks if John has ever given a sperm sample before. Jane admits she doesn't know. The doctor then gives Jane a requisition for a semen analysis and the name of a reproductive endocrinologist who is *not* a gynecologist. "Tell John to go to any lab to deliver this sample," he says. "In the meantime, here's the name of a doctor I know well who specilizes in fertility workups. It may take some time to get an appointment, so you may want to set it up soon. Just tell him I sent you. I'll call you if the sperm sample comes back abnormal."

Jane leaves the office and goes home. She hands the requisition over to John. John is furious. "Are you *kidding*! I'm not going to masturbate in some lab unless I *have* to! *You're* the one who wants to get checked out, so *you* get checked out! I'll deliver the sample after you're done!"

Jane feels, for lack of a better word, impotent. She doesn't want to waste her breath (and more time) waiting for John to "come around." She decides to proceed with the workup alone. When her gynecologist notices that no sperm sample for John has come in, he assumes no news is good news. Perhaps they decided against going ahead with the workup? Perhaps she conceived? He doesn't follow up with her regarding the sperm sample (it's really not his responsibility.)

Now, three months later, Jane is meeting with the reproductive endocrinologist.

DOCTOR: Hello, Jane. I'm Dr. Smith. I understand you want to get pregnant.
JANE: That's right.

DOCTOR: Are you married? (Translation: Where's your partner?)
JANE: Yes I am. (Translation: Maybe John should have come with me.)

DOCTOR: Are you healthy otherwise? (Translation: Have you been screened for any STDs or health problems that are dangerous to a pregnancy?)
JANE: Yes. (Translation: I don't know.)

DOCTOR: Does your husband have a clean bill of health? (Translation: Was his semen analysis normal?)
JANE: Yes, he does. (Translation: I don't know.)

DOCTOR: How long have you been trying to get pregnant? (Translation: How long have you been having frequent intercourse during ovulation?)
JANE: Two years. (Translation: We've been having unprotected sex for two years—when we've felt like it.)

DOCTOR: Are your cycles regular? (Translation: Are you ovulating?)
JANE: Well, I get my period regularly, if that's what you mean. (Translation: I have no idea when I'm ovulating. My periods are so irregular I gave up keeping track. But I won't tell him.)

DOCTOR: Jane, what I'd like to do is take your medical history and review your ovulation chart. (Translation: I need to see proof that you've really been "trying.")

JANE: What's an ovulation chart? (Translation: We haven't been trying.)

DOCTOR: I need to see a calendar or something where you've been marking down the days you ovulate. Those are the days you should be having intercourse. Didn't you bring one? (Translation: Are you wasting my time?)

JANE: Well, we've been having sex a few times a week for the last two years. Isn't that enough? (Translation: I haven't done any reading on fertility awareness.)

DOCTOR: I see. In that case, here's what we'll do: Sandy, my nurse, will give you a basal body thermometer test kit, and a special ovulation chart/calendar. She'll walk you through all the steps in using the kit properly. Then, come back in six months, or once the chart is filled out for six consecutive cycles. At that point I'll review the chart and do a pelvic exam and a complete medical history. Otherwise, we're just going to waste a whole lot of time and effort. (Translation: Get out of my office, go home and "try." Come back when you can *prove* you have a problem. Don't waste any more of my time.)

Jane leaves the office feeling frustrated. (Six months? By then she'll be almost 35!)

A *post-mortem*

Jane and John are definitely fertility deadbeats. They did not go for their preconception screenings and were not united as a couple. John made it seem as though Jane had the problem, and he was not willing to participate in the workup. Had John cooperated and delivered the sperm sample, Jane's *first* gynecologist would have called back. Why? Because the sperm sample would have shown that John has chlamydia (his lack of condom use exposed him to it years ago). That means Jane has chlamydia too, and may even have scarring on her fallopian tubes or *salpingitis* (inflamed fallopian tubes) from undiagnosed pelvic inflammatory disease (PID). Instead of spending six months observing her ovulation, both she and John could have been treated for chlamydia, and Jane's tubes could have been evaluated. In this time frame, microsurgery may even have been recommended to repair her tubes.

But none of this is happening. Instead, valuable time is being lost. John and Jane will spend *at least* a year going in the wrong diagnostic direction. Worse, since Jane's reproductive endocrinologist isn't a gynecologist, it may take him longer to diagnose her chlamydia. By the time he does, it may then be too late because the chlamydia may have already progressed to severe PID, leaving Jane with unsalvageable tubal damage. But here's the icing on the cake: Even if Jane's chlamydia is discovered and treated, since she lied about John's clean bill of health to begin with, John may not be treated for the chlamydia and may reinfect Jane after she *is* treated.

The Right Way to Use a Fertility Doctor

Infertility is not a disease in the sense that your life is threatened if you don't get treatment. Because of this, when you don't follow a doctor's recommendations, the doctor won't be chasing you down. That's why Jane's gynecologist didn't bother calling about the undelivered sperm sample. And if that reproductive endocrinologist never hears from Jane again, he won't be worried. Neither John's life nor Jane's is in any danger without an infertility investigation.

Alan and Cheryl Smith are the model couple when it comes to investigating infertility. They have exactly the same medical/sexual history as John and Jane, are the same age, have been married the same number of years, have also been trying since their honeymoon, and are also not getting pregnant. But they're united. Alan and Cheryl make an appointment—as a couple—with their family doctor (a family physician). Whether they realize it or not, they've just hired a "weed doctor."

DOCTOR: So, you two want to get pregnant. Have either of you been referred for preconception counseling before?

CHERYL: Can you ask us that again—in *English*?
(General laughter.)

DOCTOR: Have you been screened for any health problems or medical conditions that may be dangerous to a pregnancy?

ALAN: I haven't—have you, Cheryl?

CHERYL: Well, other than my annual Pap smear and internal exams, I don't think so.

DOCTOR: OK, then! Let's first do your screenings, and then we'll see what *that* turns up. I also want to go through your medical histories with you. Or, you can take a blank history chart and fill it out at home. Sometimes the questions are a little embarrassing, and you may also need a little more time to answer them. Now, Cheryl, I'm assuming your cycles are regular?

CHERYL: I brought along my daytimer that shows when we've had sex and when I've had my periods. We've been aiming for the middle of the cycle.

DOCTOR: I'll have a look at that, and then I may want to get you do a basal body temperature chart, which is a little more accurate. But let's not worry about that *now*. Let's do the screenings first. After all the tests are in, we can discuss Cheryl's ovulation pattern and get you two going on the right schedule.

ALAN: So you don't think we need to see a fertility specialist?

DOCTOR: Not just yet. There are quite a few tests I want to run before I decide if you have to go elsewhere. And Alan, I'll need to get a sperm sample from you.

ALAN: Can I give you a sample after you've checked out Cheryl?

DOCTOR: Nope. You first. Any tests that Cheryl goes through will be more invasive and complicated. So let's clear away any problems with you first before I send you on for a female workup.

ALAN: Can I do it at home?

DOCTOR: Sure can. Just make sure you read the instructions on the kit, and get the sample to the lab within a half hour after ejaculation.

By asking the doctor questions and being honest about what they have or *haven't* done so far, Alan and Cheryl are off to a great start. Alan also feels more comfortable and reassured about giving a sperm sample because he's heard the explanation for the sample from the *doctor* rather than relying on Cheryl's memory. He also asks questions that Cheryl may not have asked had she gone herself. They go home and do their medical history lesson, both revealing a colorful sexual history and years of unprotected sex with different partners. This tells the doctor to check for STDs *immediately* before doing anything else. He does. And, like John and Jane, Alan's semen analysis shows that he has chlamydia. Jane is checked for chlamydia too, and tests positive. The family doctor puts both Alan and Cheryl on the antibiotic *doxycycline* for ten days, counseling them about condom use until they're retested. Two weeks later, he takes a second semen sample from Alan and rechecks Cheryl. *Now* watch what happens:

DOCTOR: The antibiotics worked, and you're both "all clear" of STDs.

CHERYL: Should we go ahead and try again, like you said before?

DOCTOR: Not just yet. Cheryl, even though you didn't have any symptoms of chlamydia and felt well, your fallopian tubes may have some scarring as a result of the infection. To be honest, I think it's a waste of time for you to begin trying to conceive until we check the condition of your tubes. However, I'm not qualified to assess them. I'm going to refer you to Dr. Susan Stern. She's a gynecologist who specializes in reproductive endocrinology and fertility microsurgery.

ALAN: What about me? Who should I be seeing?

DOCTOR: Your semen analysis came back normal. You're fine. If, and I mean if, there's a problem, Cheryl's the one who will need to go for more tests and possible treatment. I'm going to make an appointment for both of you with Dr. Stern, and recommend that you see her together. She'll take it from there.

CHERYL: What if we don't like her?

DOCTOR: Come see me again, and I'll recommend some other specialists in the same field.

Alan and Cheryl are in terrific shape. They've been referred to the right specialist, who will check for any structural damage to Cheryl's tubes by doing a test called an *hysterosalpingogram* (see chapter 5). They also won't be wasting any of this specialist's precious time because their histories will be sent along to her by their primary care physician before they get there. She'll be able to review their charts at her leisure without doing any of the annoying guesswork that Jane's specialist had to. Then, if all goes well, Alan and Cheryl will start to officially "try." By doing it this way, they're getting to the bottom of their fertility problem much faster. As for John and Jane, they'll try for another six months and possibly longer without anyone treating their chlamydia. By then, Jane's tubes may become damaged beyond repair.

Once you are referred to the right specialist, it's important to know how to maximize your visits. Here are some guidelines:

1. *Tape record your visit.* Specialists often say a lot in a small space of time. When you're upset or overwhelmed by all of the information being hurled at you, you often don't hear what the specialist is saying. Tape recording the visit is helpful because you can replay information when you're more relaxed and can better understand what you've been told.

2. *Take a list of questions with you, and tape record the answers.* When you have a lot of questions, make a list so you don't forget them. The specialist has an obligation to answer all of your questions, and if he or she doesn't have time, there are some options. Give the

doctor your list and ask if he or she can address your questions in your next appointment. If that's not possible, agree on a time when the specialist can call you at home. As a final resort, ask if there is a resident studying with the specialist with whom you can arrange a question-and-answer session. (Usually, any resident—a "specialist in training"—can answer your questions.)

3. *Request literature or videos on your condition from the specialist, or get the number of an organization you can call for more information.*

4. *If it's relevant, ask the specialist to draw you a diagram of the problem. For example, for many structural problems, these diagrams often involve "plumbing" analogies that can instantly communicate the problem.*

The Patient's Bill of Rights

In the past, doctors were expected to be godlike creatures, while patients were expected to play passive roles. This kind of doctor-patient relationship doesn't exist anymore. We are now consumers of health care. We've gone from patient to impatient. We want results; we want *value* for our money. Whether we live in the United States or Canada, the patient is the customer—the one who ultimately pays the doctor's salary. (Canadians pay for health care with their taxes.) As a result, the doctor-patient relationship is now a two-way street, not unlike a marriage. What do you have a right to expect from a doctor?

- *As much information as you want.* This means that you have every right to know your diagnosis, prognosis (your doctor's estimate of when you'll get better), alternate forms of treatment, your doctor's recommendations, and the basis of his or her recommendations (i.e., research studies, hunch, etc.).

- *Time to address questions and concerns.* If your doctor doesn't have time to answer questions, you should be able to call him or her or make another appointment that serves as a question-and-answer period.

- *Reasonable access.* You and your doctor must decide together what *reasonable* means. Do you need weekly, quarterly, or annual appointments? Or do you just want to see the doctor when you feel like it? How much advance booking time do you need to get an appointment?

- *Participation in the decision-making process.* To do this, you'll have to ask questions and be willing to educate yourself about your condition (i.e., request literature from your doctor, etc.).

- *Adequate emergency care and the right to know your doctor's substitute.* Who looks after you after hours, or when your doctor is sick or on vacation? Is there a substitute doctor?
- *To know who has access to your health records.* How confidential are your health records? Can your doctor release them to just anyone—your employer, insurance companies, government authorities? What are your doctor's legal obligations with respect to health records, and what are yours?
- *To know what it costs.* If you live in the United States, you have the right to know what your bill is in advance. Get an estimate and have the doctor break down each charge so you know exactly what you're paying for and what your insurance plan is covering. If you live in Canada, make sure all appointments, tests, and procedures are covered by your Province before you consent to anything.
- *The right to be seen on time.* If you're on time for an appointment, your doctor should be as well. Do you generally have to wait more than 30 minutes in the reception area before your doctor sees you?
- *To change doctors.* Yes, you can fire your doctor. If you're unhappy with your current doctor, or simply need a change, you have every right to switch. Make sure you arrange for your records to be transferred. NOTE: Before you switch, you may want to arrange to meet with your current doctor to discuss your reasons for changing.
- *A second opinion, or a consultation with a specialist.* If your doctor can't make an adequate diagnosis, you can insist on a referral to either another doctor or a specialist.

The Infertility Patient's Bill of Rights

Because infertility workups and treatments are so complex and involved, an infertility patient also has the right to:
- get respect from all medical staff;
- have his or her feelings validated by all medical staff;
- be informed about all the steps involved in investigation and treatment, the *order* in which each test will be performed, the *realistic* time frame involved, and all the risks and side effects of tests and treatments;
- have all the facts regarding treatment outlined: the steps involved, number of cycles involved, success rates, and possible risks and side effects; and
- appropriate tax information in case you can claim some of your expenses on your next tax return.

The Doctor's Bill of Rights

Remember, it's a two-way street. Your doctor has an unwritten bill of rights, too. Just as you're entitled to certain information and courtesies, so is your doctor. What exactly does your doctor have the right to expect from you?

- *Full disclosure.* Doctors aren't telepathic. If you're hiding information (certain family or medical history, prescriptions, addictions, allergies, eating disorders, specific symptoms), it's unfair to expect an accurate diagnosis. What if your doctor prescribes a drug that you're allergic to or one that conflicts with your other medication?

- *Common courtesy.* Treat your doctor like a business associate. If you make an appointment, show up; if you need to cancel, give 24 hours' notice.

- *Advance planning.* Plan your visit in advance and think carefully about your symptoms. Don't just go to your doctor with a vague complaint such as "I'm not feeling well" and expect a full diagnosis. When you make an appointment, tell the receptionist how much time you think you'll need for a full examination, and write down your symptoms. Give the doctor something to work with.

- *Questions and interruptions.* If you don't understand something, ask. Interrupt the doctor if necessary and ask for simpler explanations. If you don't do this, you can't blame your doctor for not giving you enough information.

- *Follow advice and follow through.* Take medication as directed and follow advice. That's what you're paying the doctor for. If you're experiencing side effects, if you have a problem with his or her advice, or if your condition has worsened as a result of the advice, let the doctor know. Full disclosure strikes again.

- *No harassment.* If you have a problem, go through reasonable channels; dial the after-hours emergency number the doctor leaves with the answering service, or call your doctor's office during business hours. Don't continuously call the doctor at home at four in the morning, and don't call the office ten times a day with every little ache and pain.

- *Enough time to make a diagnosis.* Diagnoses don't happen overnight. Allow the doctor enough time to examine you and run the necessary tests. Don't expect miracles in 15 minutes. This might mean that you need to wait longer for an appointment so your doctor can schedule enough time to fully examine you.

- *Room for disagreement.* What you think is in your best interests may not be what your doctor thinks is best. Allow for a difference of opinion and give your doctor a chance to explain his or her side. Don't just leave in a huff and threaten to sue. Maybe your doctor is right.

- *Professional conduct.* Don't request unusual favors that compromise your doctor's moral beliefs, and don't ask your doctor to do something illegal (i.e., writing bogus notes to your employer so you can claim disability pay.)

Incidentally, if even a few of these "rights" are abused, your doctor has the right to resign as your doctor and request that you seek care elsewhere.

When to Get a Second Opinion

When it comes to fertility treatment, getting a second opinion is often a necessary route, which translates into seeing two separate doctors about the same set of symptoms. The doctors can be in the same field or specialize in different areas. This can happen at either the diagnostic or treatment stage of an infertility investigation. It's difficult to know whether you're justified in getting a second opinion. Just because you don't like the sound of your diagnosis doesn't mean you *require* another opinion. Let's say your doctor suspects that your infertility is caused by endometriosis and wants to perform a laparoscopy procedure to confirm his or her suspicions. You might not like the sound of this and decide to see a holistic doctor or an herbalist instead, who may tell you that you're under stress and only need to rest and take various herbs in order to conceive. Of course, this is a much more soothing diagnosis, but in this case your doctor is the one who is right.

The following guidelines should help you decide whether a second opinion is warranted. If you answer yes to even one of the questions below, you're probably justified in seeking a second opinion.

1. *Is the diagnosis uncertain?* If your doctor can't find out what's wrong or isn't sure whether he of she is correct, you have every right to go elsewhere.
2. *Is the diagnosis life-threatening?* In this case, hearing the same news from someone else may help you cope better with your illness or come to terms with the diagnosis. Diagnoses like cancer, however, usually won't change; the diagnosis is based on carefully analyzed test results, not just on the patient's symptoms.
3. *Is the treatment controversial, experimental, or risky?* You might not question the diagnosis but have problems with the recommended treatment, such as certain potent fertility drugs or microsurgical procedures. If you're not comfortable with the recommended treatment, perhaps another doctor can recommend a different approach.
4. *Is the treatment not working?* This is a real dilemma for fertility patients. If you've been in

treatment for a reasonable length of time (see in chapter 10), and you're not conceiving, maybe the wrong diagnosis was made, or perhaps the treatment recommended is not right for you. Seeing another doctor may help to confirm or alleviate concerns.

5. *Are risky tests or procedures being recommended?* If you don't like the sound of microsurgery, hearing it from someone else might make you accept the procedure more readily. Or, you may find out that microsurgery is premature and isn't necessary after all. Find out if there are alternate therapies or procedures that can yield the same results.

6. *Do you want another approach?* A 45-year-old woman who is entering menopause wants to prolong her fertility with fertility drugs so she can conceive. Her doctor refuses to treat her, saying that she's too old to have a child. The woman finds this approach unacceptable and sees a second doctor who *doesn't* have a problem with her age and is willing to put her on the drugs for a limited period of time.

7. *Is the doctor competent?* If you suspect your doctor is incompetent, seek a second opinion either to reaffirm your faith in him or her or to confirm your original suspicions.

Heal Thyself

When you're investigating or treating infertility, there's a lot you need to know when it comes to choosing the right combination of doctors and making sure you're receiving the best care possible. There are also a number of ways you can heal yourself during the investigative or treatment phase of your fertility problem.

1. Educate yourself. Learn about the physical, psychological and emotional processes involved with conception and pregnancy.

2. Learn about all your options, and choose the practitioners appropriate for you.

3. Inform yourself about hospital policies and regulations that will affect your treatment and possible pregnancy.

4. Arrange for a companion or support person to help you through your treatment if your partner is unavailable.

5. Calmly and clearly make your preferences known to your doctors regarding testing, alternative therapies, or objections to certain procedures at the beginning of your treatment.

6. Research the costs of your treatment in advance. (Canadians will need to find out what treatments are covered by the Province.)

7. Notify your practitioners if you intend to seek care elsewhere, or intend to stop treatment.

Much of the information you'll need to fulfill this list is provided throughout the book. Moving on to the "trying" phase of the process may happen immediately after you've been screened for various health problems or have been treated for one. Before you begin charting the rhythms of your individual menstrual cycle, it's important to be aware of how certain lifestyle habits can interfere with infertility. In other words, you and your partner should go through the exercise of evaluating whether your own *habits* are creating a barrier to conception.

The Seven Habits of Highly Infertile People

One of the major differences between couples in the 1960s and couples today is that both partners usually need to be in the workforce in order to make ends meet. In many cases, this translates into two-car families; long commutes to and from work; poor eating habits as a result of skipped breakfasts; fast-food lunches and dinners; and intense physical workouts to stay in shape. To combat the stress and fatigue, most of us indulge in a few bad habits, such as gulping coffee, smoking, and drinking alcohol. Many of us will also take over-the-counter medications to fight off headaches, fatigue, and other side effects of stress. For women, these habits can mean interrupted ovulation cycles, skipped periods, and decreased libidos; for men, these habits can mean decreased sperm counts, decreased libidos, and, in extreme cases, bouts of impotence.

Your own lifestyle habits can have a powerful influence on your fertility. "Get more sleep, more rest, and eat right" are the usual words of advice. It's not enough. This chapter is devoted to outlining *all* the lifestyle habits that can affect a couple's fertility. Obviously, when there *is* a hormonal imbalance or structural problem at work, changing your lifestyle probably will not help you conceive. But when you're planning conception, and no delay is identified at the "weeding," it's crucial to assess whether your lifestyle is "fertility friendly" to *begin* with *before* you undergo an expensive workup or begin charting your fertility cycle. To continue the yardwork analogy from chapter 1: you've pulled the weeds, now you need to prepare the *soil*. Too much sun, too much water, or too little of each can profoundly affect your garden. You also need to assess whether your soil has any *contaminants*. This chapter serves as your lifestyle "checklist" and discusses seven common, not-so-healthy habits.

1. Bad Habits

Whether you smoke, drink coffee and/or alcohol, or use addictive drugs such as marijuana or other narcotics, your vice(s) could certainly affect your current or future fertility. The traditional thinking was that only *women* needed to purify their bodies, which most women do once they discover they're pregnant. But few couples realize the importance of purifying their systems *prior* to conception, and even fewer understand how important it is for *both* partners to rid themselves of these indulgences when planning a pregnancy. So here's the bad news about your bad habits . . .

Women

Much has been written about alcohol use during pregnancy and the risks of fetal alcohol syndrome. As a result, very few women who educate themselves about prenatal care will choose to drink during pregnancy. Unfortunately, very few women understand how alcohol can affect them in the "trying-to-get-pregnant" phase, which can be equally hazardous.

Even moderate drinking (one to two glasses of wine per week, for example) can increase the level of the hormone *prolactin*. Prolactin is the hormone responsible for milk production after pregnancy. It does this by suppressing the levels of estrogen and progesterone in your body, which, in turn, will suppress ovulation. This is why breastfeeding has been touted as a natural contraceptive, although it is by *no* means 100% effective. If, however, your prolactin levels are too high *prior* to conception, your ovulation cycle can go haywire and you will have difficulty conceiving. (See chapter 3 for more details about the ovulation cycle.) In extreme cases, a condition known as *hyperprolactinemia* (meaning "too much prolactin") can set in, which will render a woman infertile until the problem is corrected.

Alcohol isn't the only drug that can increase prolactin levels. Antidepressant medications (which may be prescribed), painkillers (for headaches, menstrual cramps and so on), and hallucinogens such as marijuana have all been cited as substances that can cause hyperprolactinemia.

As for smoking, more women die from lung cancer than any other disease, and women who smoke greatly increase their chances of developing other kinds of cancers (breast, gynecological, colon). Furthermore, smoking significantly reduces a woman's fertility. *No one knows exactly why this is.* The current theory is that smoking "pollutes" all of your reproductive organs and reproductive system, affecting overall job performance. Different studies point to reduced levels of estrogen and poor cervical mucus, higher tendencies to develop pelvic infections, and subsequent tubal damage. Worse, high levels of nicotine, which can be found in cervical mucus, can be toxic to your partner's sperm. To date, all studies that tracked the effect of smoking on female fertility came to the same conclusion: More women who smoke are infertile than are women who *don't* smoke. As for the hazards of smoking in early pregnancy, the list includes an increased risk of ectopic pregnancy and miscarriage (both discussed in chapter 9).

Finally, women who drink coffee or other caffeinated beverages and who are trying to get pregnant may want to start eliminating caffeine altogether. A recent study by the U.S. National Institute of Environmental Health Sciences found that the more caffeine a woman consumes, the less likely she is to conceive. In fact, women who drank the equivalent of one cup of brewed coffee per day were found to be half as likely to conceive as women who had no caffeine. Don't panic, though. The study also found that the effects of caffeine on female fertility are *short-term*. If you drank six cups of coffee a day two years ago and have since given up caffeine, you will be just as likely to conceive now as you woul if you had no history of caffeine consumption.

For women coping with infertility, cutting out their vices may be easier said than done. Here's a typical scenario: A woman has intercourse mid-cycle and suddenly "purifies" herself in anticipation of conception. Instead of her anxiously awaited feelings of nausea and morning sickness, she gets PMS and then her period—a scarlet reminder of another "failed" cycle. Feeling frustrated and angry, she ties one on and gets good and drunk. Or, she may decide to start smoking again in a what-does-it-matter-now rationale. All in all, a vicious cycle.

Men

Male fertility is also affected by smoking, alcohol, and recreational drugs. It's believed that nicotine reduces testosterone levels by altering the *Leydig cell*, the cell that produces testosterone. This can cause low sperm counts, poor motility, and an increase in abnormal sperm (two heads, no tail, deformed tails). One Greek-American joint study found that men who smoked more than twenty cigarettes per day had significant defects in the tails of their sperm. Research also shows that that cigarette smoke adversely affects the overall male reproductive tract, causing the tissues and tubules responsible for smooth sperm production to operate in a type of "smog" that reduces fertility. Finally, strong anecdotal evidence has found long-term infertility to be suddenly "cured" when the male partners stop smoking.

Alcohol consumption in men can lead to poor sperm quality, poor libido, and even impotence. As alcohol damages the liver, estrogen levels rise, which counteracts testosterone levels normally responsible for libido and sperm quality. High estrogen levels in men are linked only to long-term, heavy alcohol use, however. One beer or alcoholic beverage a day will most likely *not* cause high estrogen levels or interfere with male fertility. No one is sure, though, what constitutes "heavy" alcohol use in men. One British infertility expert suggests that the daily maximum limit for men should be no more than two to three pints of beer, which is equal to one-half bottle of wine, or two to three shots of hard liquor. Of course, even if a man does not go over his daily allowable "maximum," any amount of intoxication will significantly affect his ability to sustain an erection and hence father a child.

Marijuana, barbiturates, and other narcotics are a different story. Sperm quality is affected by heavy and/or frequent marijuana use. Essentially, the sperm get "stoned" and are not able to swim as well or move as effectively (motility) up the female reproductive tract. Marijuana may also increase the number of abnormal sperm produced. As for other recreational drugs, they interfere more with performance than with sperm quality, causing impotence and various ejaculatory disorders.

2. Coping Habits

Coping with the stress of daily existence can have adverse affects on both female and male fertility. Most women have experienced at least one fouled-up menstrual cycle because of job or personal stress. (Ironically, for teens and younger women, missing periods because of stress is most often caused by worrying about being pregnant!) Similarly, most men have experienced at least one bout of impotence or ejaculatory problems that is stress related. When men *can* perform sexually under great stress, their sperm counts are actually reduced. Stress-related situations revolve around career changes, job loss, death in the family, moving, exams, stressful workloads, and emotional upheavals.

Under stress, the hypothalamus, which controls both the female and male hormonal cycles (see chapters 3 and 4) functions more slowly. This slows down the pituitary gland, which in turn slows down the sex hormones of either the stressed-out man or woman. This translates into either a missed period or a decreased sperm count. It's not really understood *why* this happens, but it is considered a protective mechanism, a sort of prehistoric parachute in the human body. The body senses the stress levels and decides to stop either ovulation or sperm production for that month preventing a "stressed" pregnancy. This protective mechanism isn't unique to humans; animals in cramped quarters in either laboratories or zoos often cannot be able to reproduce.

Currently, fertility experts assume that between 5–10% of all infertility is stress-related. Translation: Stress is a factor in 5-10% of all persons with either irregular menstrual cycles or reduced sperm counts.

"Just Relax . . . "

We hear these frustrating words often from friends, relatives, or even doctors. *There's no such thing as trying to "relax" when your life is stressful.* In fact, under stressful circumstances, you should listen to your *body* and *not* try to force conception.

Finding a strategic method for coping with stress is a expansive topic that drives a good portion of the how-to book and seminar market. The strategy that works for you is *highly* individualized, so what you find helpful, your partner may not. Consult the resource list at the back of this book for more information on relaxation books, methods, and therapists. To indicate how powerful some of these methods can be, a clinical study published in a 1991 issue of *Fertility and Sterility* revealed some amazing statistics. The study compared conception rates of two groups of infertile women. Seventeen percent of the women who had only medical treatment conceived, whereas 35% of the women who underwent a specific program of meditation, exercise, and yoga, *in addition to medical treatment*, conceived. In short, adding this particular relaxation method to medical treatments doubled these women's chances of conception. It's important to realize that the underlying cause of your stress may pass with time, as is the case with a death, a job change, a move, and so on.

When your stress is clearly job related, there are a number of ways you can minimize your stress, which are discussed in the Work Habits section. Sometimes the only solution is to change either your job or your career if you want to lead a more stress-free life.

Guidelines for Seeking Help

Many of us cope with stress by indulging in some of the bad habits discussed above, or overdoing it in the exercise or eating departments. When this happens, your fertility becomes even more threatened as your lifestyle becomes *more* unhealthy. Whether your stress is a short-term or long-term problem, there are certain situations that warrant counseling. In fact, if you recognize yourself in any of the following statements, going for counseling is a good idea.

1. I need a few drinks every day (wine, beer, liquor, etc.) just to unwind.
2. I need to take drugs (cocaine, marijuana) in order to cope.

3. I pig out when I'm under stress and then punish myself with a really intense workout.

4. I'm losing interest in activities I used to enjoy (including sexual activities).

5. I'm not sleeping well. I wake up very early and can't seem to get back to sleep.

6. I feel very sad and depressed and haven't been able to pinpoint why.

7. I have no appetite; it's a struggle just to eat.

8. I'm always sleepy. I seem to need constant sleep just to function.

9. I'm very irritable and anxious over issues that never bothered me before (partner's habits, etc.).

Finally, if you have a history of psychiatric illness (manic/bipolar depression, biologic depression, schizophrenia) or have a family history of psychiatric illness (which means that you're more likely to develop a psychiatric disorder yourself), you should make sure that the stress you're suffering is indeed from an external source and not a symptom of a psychiatric illness. In some cases, you may require medications, many of which can control disorders related to brain chemistry imbalances (such as numerous forms of biologic depression). If you're already on medication to control a previously diagnosed psychiatric disorder, and you're feeling stressed, make sure you have your medication dosages adjusted accordingly. Newer antidepressant medications (developed in the late 1980s and early 1990s) should not interfere with your fertility, but some of the older medications developed in the 1960s and 1970s may have some nasty side effects. Discuss the risks of any antidepressant medications you're taking with your primary care doctor or psychiatrist.

3. Eating Habits

When your eating habits are unhealthy, the worst hit your body may take is below the belt. Both male and female fertility is dependent on healthy diets and stable weights. Because of the culture we live in, women are more susceptible to eating disorders than men, but sperm count can also be lowered through obesity or underweight (see the "Men" section below).

Women

When it comes to true obesity, most women do not become obese until they begin dieting! Only a tiny portion of women are obese because of truly hereditary factors. Most women who think they are overweight are actually at an *ideal* weight for their height and body size. There is a crippling fear of obesity in Western society. Sixty percent of young girls develop distorted body images between grades one and six and believe that they are "fat," and 70% of all women begin dieting between the ages of 14 and 21. This just isn't healthy. A 1991 documentary reported that most women, when given a choice, would rather be dead than fat!

Eating disorders are so widespread that abnormal patterns of eating are becoming accepted in the general population. Some parents that are actually *starving* their young daughters in an effort to keep them thin. The two most common eating disorders involve starvation dieting (in extreme cases, this develops into *anorexia nervosa*) and binging followed by purging (eating copious amounts of food, and then self-inducing vomiting or abusing laxatives, known as *bulimia*). Perhaps the most accepted abnormal dieting conduct revolves around overexercising, discussed later in this chapter, which has spawned a new term: exercise bulimics. Generally, all women have displayed or will display some type of abnormal eating behavior. At the minimal level, women often will not eat one day prior to a fancy function in an effort to fit into their outfit, or "look thinner." Other women will binge/purge by abusing laxatives and diuretics. Many women will define "binging" as eating three well-balanced meals in one day, instead of the usual no-breakfast/salad-for-lunch/salad-for-dinner routine.

The truth is, living in fear of obesity can be more dangerous to your health than being 25–30 pounds overweight, the technical definition of obese. Most women have a desired weight goal set at roughly 10 pounds *under* their ideal weight; many women who think they are overweight are either at an ideal weight or 10 pounds *underweight*. Women need to relearn their eating habits, understand why they gain weight when they starve themselves, understand the *reproductive* hazards of eating disorders, and reprogram their body image to welcome normal, necessary body fat.

Starvation diets, purging and binging rituals, and yo-yo dieting affect ovulation. If you have difficulty eating regularly or normally, you need to see a nutritionist to get your diet under control. Unless you're eating balanced meals and are maintaining a *stable* weight, you won't be creating optimum conditions for conception. When the female body is malnourished, it stops ovulating because it can't sustain a pregnancy. One doctor told me about an aboriginal tribe in Australia that has developed a unique protective mechanism: Women of that particular tribe menstruate only at certain times of the year, when the food cycle is abundant. During World War II, up to 50% of the women who were in concentration camps stopped menstruating within two months after their capture.

When you are truly starving, the body's ability to adapt to adverse conditions is amazing. But when you're jumping back and forth between starving and eating normally, you'll most certainly gain weight. Here's why: Your body is very smart. When it doesn't get enough calories, it gets tougher and more efficient. When you starve yourself, it *learns how to function on less calories*. When you go back to eating normally or eating less than you ate before you started dieting, you'll gain weight! Your body will be jarred by the sudden calorie intake and store it as fat for "later" when the "famine" strikes again. As far as your body is concerned, it doesn't know that you're living in North America and can have food anytime you want. Your body is trying to save you, not do you in! So be good to it. The gynecological consequences of starvation diets and yo-yo dieting are irregular cycles or even long bouts of amenorrhea (discussed in chapter 3), which translates into infertility; boneloss during pregnancy and before menopause (which creates huge problems during and after menopause), and future ovarian problems. Starving yourself results in the cruelest of "vicious cycles": Unless you keep reducing your food intake until you *do* starve to death, you'll gain weight to the extent of becoming *overweight*.

How much food should you eat?

The average nonpregnant woman in her childbearing years requires about 1,680 calories a day to maintain the right energy balance and ideal weight. This is an appropriate amount of calories, assuming that your food absorption, gastric emptying, secretion of digestive juices, and motility of your digestive tract are all intact. Conditions that affect all these elements are:

- weight changes (sudden weight loss, yo-yo dieting, or sudden weight gain);
- diarrhea (often caused by abusing laxatives);
- mild or severe anemia (often caused by heavy periods; see chapter 3);
- diuretics (nutrients are taken out of the blood and excreted in the urine);
- thyroid disorders (your metabolism may speed up or slow down depending on the disorder);
- lactose intolerance (interferes with a high-calcium diet);
- diabetes;
- HIV; and
- high cholesterol, hypertension, and heart problems;

The above is only a sample of the unique problems that can affect the dietary needs of each woman. The only way to meet dietary requirements is to tailor your food and vitamin intake to your weight, height, culture, medical history, and lifestyle. How do you do this? Request a referral to a nutritionist. All hospitals have nutritionists on staff, and all doctors have lists of nutritionists they can refer you to.

When you meet with your nutritionist, put together a realistic food plan that you can stick to. If you have gained weight, you should be able to lose it by eating sensibly and following your food plan. Stay away from quick-fix diets, and try to set practical goals such as losing 1–2 pounds a week instead of 5–10. Eating healthy will also help improve the efficiency of any medications you're taking, because your digestive system will be better able to absorb them. For many women, consulting a therapist to deal with an eating disorder is a more appropriate route. Your primary care physician can refer you to one.

If you truly are obese

If you're overweight by at least 25–30 pounds, (i.e., 25–30 pounds over your medically ideal weight—*not* your desired weight), your ovulation cycle can also be affected. Estrogen is stored in fat cells, which is one reason why overweight women tend to be at risk for certain estrogen-dependent cancers such as breast, endometrial, ovarian, or colon. The fat cells convert fat into estrogen, creating a type of estrogen reserve that may interfere with ovulation. Slimming down to a more ideal weight *with the help of a qualified nutritionist* not only may put your ovulation cycles back on track, but will also help you acheive a healthier lifestyle.

Finally, the weight may interfere with intercourse positions, which naturally will have a bearing on your fertility. Usually, though, weight-affected sexual performance is more of a problem for obese men than for women.

Men

Although women in Western culture are more prone to starving themselves, men are more prone to (and even encouraged to) overeat. This can spell trouble for male fertility. The fat cells store androgen (a collection of male hormones that *includes* testosterone), just as fat cells store estrogen in women. But the fat cells in males can *convert* androgen into estrogen, causing overweight men to develop breast tissue (we've all seen this before, thinking it's just fat) and even a more feminine complexion, with softer skin and less facial hair. All this boils down to reduced testosterone levels and a dramatically reduced sperm count.

Obese men will also have more trouble with sexual performance. For example, excess weight in the abdominal area may get in the way of inserting the penis high enough inside the vagina; unless the sperm is ejaculated well inside the vagina, the sperm cannot swim as effectively up the cervix and female reproductive tract. Other problems may involve intercourse comfort and positioning. The man's weight may interfere with his own and/or his partner's sexual comfort, causing premature ejaculation, premature or involuntary withdrawal, or inadequate stimulation to maintain an erection.

Males who are overweight should get down to a stable weight through the help of a qualified nutritionist and a primary care physician. In some cases, an underactive thyroid may be the cause of a sudden weight gain. In addition to fertility problems, men who are obese are at a higher risk of developing heart problems, strokes, and various kinds of cancers.

Underweight men may also experience decreased libido and sperm counts. Infertility has been seen among men who are 25% below their medically ideal body weights. In Western culture, underweight men are generally a rare commodity, seen only in conjunction with chronic illnesses such as colitis or with more life-threatening illnesses such as cancer or AIDS. Achieving underweight is never a *deliberate* goal among men the way it is among women. Persistent weight loss due to poor appetite, however, is often a symptom of biologic depression, which may require psychiatric treatment. Persistent diarrhea, perspiration, and prolonged fevers are symptoms of illnesses ranging from parasitical, bacterial, or viral infections. In some cases, sudden weight loss could also be sign of an overactive thyroid gland. Unexplained weight loss should always be followed up with a full physical.

About Those Chemicals and Pesticides . . .

There are several nutritional and medical experts who have gone on the record to say that chemically processed food is bad for your reproductive organs. They recommend avoiding food that is processed and treated or contains artificial hormones. Eating organic seasonal and local foods is a good rule to follow. The U.S. Department of Agriculture and Ministry of Food and Agriculture in Canada have consumer information lines that can direct you to stores that carry organic produce. Some nutritionists also recommend sticking to the outside aisles of a supermarket when food shopping to avoid buying an excessive amount of canned, bottled, or boxed goods.

Anne Marie Colbin, in her 1986 book *Food and Healing*, cautions women about food that involves the reproductive systems of animals or contains both natural and artificial hormones. Her list includes free-range and hormone-fed chicken eggs, as well as meat from animals raised on estrogens. Free-range animal *meat* is perfectly fine, however.

A Danish study, published in a June 1994 issue of *The Lancet*, looked into the effects of chemicals on human fertility and revealed that male organic farmers who eat pesticide-free food are able to produce roughly *double* the average number of sperm. The Danish research team maintains that this latest study seems to link pesticides and food additives to a worldwide decline in male fertility over the last half-century. The study is considered inconclusive, since only 30 men were involved in the experiment.

Watch your peas

Although I've always considered peas to be a reasonably harmless vegetable, Jean Carper, in her 1989 book *Food and Pharmacy*, claims that they're the *worst* thing you can eat when you're trying to conceive. Apparently, peas contain an antifertility chemical called *m-xylohydroquinone*, which somehow interferes with progesterone and estrogen. In fact, one of the few studies done on peas and fertility found that peas have an "oral contraceptive" property. (Definitely something the Green Giant ought to know about!)

4. Exercise Habits

Regular exercise should always accompany a healthy lifestyle, but in 1995, the definition of being "in shape" has come to mean an exaggerated physique for both men and women. For both sexes, the pressure to pump up has reproductive consequences.

Women

Rigorous, strenuous exercise has become one of the tenets of socially accepted feminine behavior in the 1990s. It's not enough to look like a concentration camp victim; women now must look like concentration camp victims with *biceps*! Strenuous exercise often accompanies an eating disorder, and together they can wreak havoc on the female hormonal cycle. The appropriate amount of exercise women require is a brisk 15-minute walk each day. Eliminating all fat from the female body and building up biceps is *not* what a healthy female body is all about; this trend has more to do with "masculinizing" the female body than "feminizing" it. While exercising and toning certainly part of a healthy lifestyle, it's important to do it for enjoyment and not because you're obsessed with maintaining a toned appearance. Overexercising can interfere with ovulation, causing women to miss their periods altogether or to experience long bouts of no periods, called amenorrhea (see chapter 3). It's not unusual for female athletes to stop menstruating when they're in training.

Exercise vs. exorcise

In an age of eating disorders, a new form of bulimia has come into vogue as women binge and then overexercise to *exorcise* the caloric demons from within. This common food/fitness perversion is a disturbing lifestyle reality for many women and may warrant the intervention of a therapist as well as a nutritionist. If you're exercising out of guilt because you think you've binged, please seek professional guidance. This is not a healthy way to exercise and can do more long-term damage than you think.

Men

Of course, the body building trends for women originated in the male gymnasium. Unfortunately, few men are immune to the allure of an Arnold Schwarzenegger body type. This has led to some unique problems for men trapped in the bodybuilding craze.

Anabolic steroids, which are on their way out of vogue for professional athletes, are still very much in use by men who want to achieve that pro-athlete look. In addition to numerous health problems, anabolic steroids can cause *long-term male infertility*. Anabolic steroids are essentially pure testosterone derivatives, which cause a *huge* increase in testosterone levels in the steroid user. Testosterone levels are controlled by both the pituitary gland and hypothalamus gland, located in the brain. (See chapters 3 and 4 for more details.) When these glands see a rise in testosterone, they send a "STOP PRODUCTION" message to the testes, believing that the testes are being overworked. As a result, the testes actually *shrink* in size, and the steroid user's natural testosterone levels dramatically drop. Even when he stops using the steroids, the user's testosterone levels can remain far lower than normal for years after use. A 22-year old male who body-builds today with the help of steroids may be in for a shock when he's 32 and suffering from low testosterone levels linked to steroids he stopped using when he was 25.

5. Personal Hygiene Habits

It's too bad our reproductive organs don't come with an owner's manual that tells us how to care and maintain all parts. Many basic hygiene habits can have a dramatic affect on both male and female fertility.

Women

As a woman, I don't have to tell you that we're prone to both vaginal and urinary tract infections. These infections not only interfere with observing your cervical mucus (see chapter 3), but will also decrease the quality of your mucus. Mucus is necessary to help the sperm swim up the female reproductive tract and fertilize the egg.

One of the worst female hygiene habits is douching. Douching rids your vagina of friendly bacteria, which is important for maintaining its ecosystem. Douching is never recommended after menstruation, even though many women practice it. As long you bathe regularly, your vagina and uterus are self-cleaning and will do everything that's necessary on their own. Finally, if you do have a bacterial or fungal infection, douching can push the bacteria or fungus higher inside your vagina, worsening the infection.

Avoid perfumes and dyes that can get into your vagina. Many of the chemicals used in these products can cause vaginal irritation and inflammation (vaginitis). Perfumes are found in many feminine products such as sprays, pads, and tampons, but you should also be careful of perfumed or colored toilet paper, hair care products that you may use in the bath or shower, certain bath or shower gels, and deodorant soaps. Here are some other hygiene tips to follow that can help prevent vaginal or urinary tract infections:

- *Avoid wearing tight clothing around your vagina.* Tight pants, panties, and nylon pantyhose prevent your vagina from breathing and make it warmer and moister for a yeast infection to develop. Wear loose pants that allow your vagina to breathe, switch to knee-highs or old-fashioned stockings, or limit your pantyhose wearing for special occasions. Go bottomless to bed to let air into your vagina.
- *Wear only 100% cotton clothing and/or natural fibers around your vagina.* Synthetic underwear and polyester pants are not good ideas. All-cotton underwear, denim, wool, or rayon pants that are loose fitting are fine.
- *Don't insert anything into a dry vagina.* Whether it's a finger, penis, or tampon, make sure your vagina is well-lubricated before insertion. Dry vaginas can be prone to abrasions during insertion, which make excellent homes for yeast.
- *Avoid long car trips on vinyl seats.* New research indicates that vinyl seats increase a woman's risk of developing a yeast infection because the vinyl traps moisture and doesn't allow the crotch area to breathe. For longer car trips, sit on a towel.
- *Urinate before and after intercourse.* Experts recommend that you empty your bladder both before and immediately after sex. Urinating after sex will also help to wash out the bacteria from the urethra. Basically, the urethra can become irritated with frequent intercourse, and more bacteria may get inside the urethra, which leads to the bladder. Many women hold back their urge to urinate during intercourse, which can aggravate matters.

A word about tampons

Most North American tampons are a rayon-cotton blend that contain a cross-section of chemicals that include dioxin residue from the chlorine bleaching process (how do you think they get them white?) and the production of rayon. Other ingredients are magnesium, boron, aluminium, litanium, surfactants, acids, alcohols, waxes, and hydrocarbons.

In the early 1980s, tampons were placed on the list of high-risk medical devices, along with intrauterine devices (IUDs) and heart pacemakers. This was in response to the toxic shock syndrome (TSS) outbreak and its association with tampons. The bottom line is that there is simply not enough information and education provided to women about the risks associated with tampons.

Toxic shock syndrome is defined as a group of symptoms. It is actually caused by bacteria already present in the vagina that adhere to the tampon. The bacteria then start producing a toxin that attacks other parts of the body. The initial symptoms of TSS are fever, nausea, vomiting, diarrhea, sore throat, and dizziness. Other symptoms include a sunburnlike rash, peeling of the skin (especially on the hands and feet), and low blood pressure. All of these symptoms are vague and can be attributed to a host of other diseases. If someone has TSS, they can easily be misdiagnosed, particularly if they have only some but not *all* of the symptoms. Currently, the list of symptoms for TSS is being revised.

Aside from TSS, there are other problems tampons can cause. Because they actively absorb menstrual blood and do not differentiate between blood and vaginal mucus, the skin that lines the vaginal walls dries up. That can lead to microulcerations and infection. Tampons should never be used between periods, during pregnancy, or when you already have a vaginal infection.

One family doctor told me that in order to practice gynecology in her office, she regularly relies on a small, surgical instrument designed to pull out old, long-forgotten tampons. Believe it or not, many women *forget* to remove their last tampon. Furthermore, many women with extremely heavy flows are in the habit of using *more than one tampon at the same time*. If you're among them, get *out* of the habit. The second one can get pushed up so high in your vagina that you can't retrieve it yourself. Change your tampon every 4–6 hours. Official warnings state that tampons left for 12–18 hours may put you at risk for TSS. Finally, remove the tampon each time you urinate to avoid infection.

A word about toilet habits

Toilet habits are one of the most common sources of bacteria in the vagina. For example, if you wipe from back to front, you could introduce fecal material into your vagina. Using a wash cloth on your vagina can transfer germs from your washcloth to your vagina. After a loose bowel movement, wet the toilet paper and clean your rectal area thoroughly so that fecal material doesn't stay on your underwear and wind up in your vagina. To prepare for less hygienic bathrooms, bring some moist wipes with you that are safe for babies' bottoms.

Men

The testicles hang below the crotch for a reason: In order for the testicles to produce enough sperm, *they need to be a few degrees cooler than normal body temperature*.

Although the "boxer shorts" story is the classic example of temperature-related infertility, this problem is more commonly seen in men who indulge in hot baths, whirlpools, or saunas. Wearing tight underwear or tight pants all the time can also reduce your sperm count, which is why boxer shorts and looser fitting pants are encouraged.

If you're exposed to an environment that has extremely hot temperatures (certain kinds of industrial plants, trapped in traffic jams with no air conditioning, etc.), your sperm count can also be reduced. Truck drivers, cab drivers, or men who sit at a desk all day are also prone to this, as well as men who live in very hot climates.

Experts suggest that cooling the testes via cool baths, ice baths, or even wearing a cool cloth inside a jock strap can dramatically improve sperm counts for temperature-related infertility.

Because your urethra is about eight inches longer than your female partner's, you're not as prone to urinary tract infections as she is, but you, too, should empty your bladder before and after intercourse (particularly after anal intercouse, which, by the way, should only be practiced with condoms), and wash your penis carefully to reduce exposure to bacteria.

6. Sexual Habits

There are some common sexual habits that can interfere with conception, but there are also common doctor-recommended "rituals" that are utterly useless in improving the odds.

Oral Sex

This first piece of news probably should go under the "Eating Habits" section. Ladies, if you're in the habit of ingesting sperm, get *out* of the habit today. Experts in the field of immunological infertility (discussed more in chapters 4, 5, 6, and 8) have found evidence suggesting that women who swallow their partners' sperm may form *antibodies* to the sperm. In a sense, swallowing the sperm is synonymous with being innoculated with it, and you could wind up giving yourself a sperm vaccine!

How is this possible? When the sperm is introduced into the digestive tract, the immune system sees it as a foreign invader, forms antibodies to it, and kills it off. Later, when the same sperm show up in the cervical canal, the immune system gets confused and attacks and kills the sperm on the spot, preventing conception. The more sperm you swallow, the more antibodies you create, so a single episode of ingesting sperm will most likely not affect your fertility. In addition, since the antibodies are created in response to one *specific* partner's sperm, past episodes of sperm swallowing with *other* partners should *not* cause your body to form antibodies to your *current* partner's sperm.

Men often ingest their own sperm when they perform cunnilingus after intercourse with their female partners. In this case, past episodes of this with other partners *can* affect your fertility today. *To avoid swallowing your own sperm, always wash your penis carefully after sex.* When a male forms antibodies to his own sperm, the antibodies may even destroy the sperm before they leave his body.

Finally, women who have anal sex with their partners should avoid getting sperm inside their rectums, which can also cause their bodies to create sperm antibodies. Anal sex may cause the tissue inside the rectum to tear, allowing the sperm easy access into the bloodstream, triggering the immune system to create antibodies.

Bear in mind that this theory is still in the research phase and has not yet been *absolutely* proven! Nevertheless, if it's true, it could be a powerful piece of preventive medicine for millions of couples.

Sexual Lubricants

Using a sexual lubricant can interfere with the sperm's survival in the vagina, as well as with the cervical mucus. If you're using a lubricant, stop.

Ejaculation Frequency

Ejaculation—in moderation—is necessary for good sperm production. Sperm that hang around too long in the *epididymis* (a section of the testicle where the sperm are stored) can spoil the bunch. In other words, dead sperm will get mixed in with live, healthy sperm and contribute to decreased sperm count. Because of this, it's important to ejaculate at least once a month through either intercourse or masturbation. However, too much ejaculation will also cause a decrease in sperm count. That's why experts recommend that couples have sex every other day around ovulation. (Some couples will have sex every other day throughout the entire cycle, which may not be realistic for those of us who work for a living!)

Many men tend to masturbate between bouts of intercourse with their partners. This is fine, but tell your partner about the frequency of your ejaculations. If you masturbated yesterday, and she's ready for sex today, it's unfair to get her hopes up. You may need to time your masturbation accordingly to allow for optimum sperm count during intercourse.

Ignore All Positioning Rituals

Planning sex around an ovulation cycle is mechanical enough, but matters are made worse by many doctors who *still* recommend the missionary position, with the woman propped up on pillows. This won't hurt, of course, *but it will not improve the odds*. Have sex any way you like. The only conditions you must meet are that the sperm be deposited deep inside the vagina. In fact, the position that turns you on the most is the one to go with; the vagina will be better lubricated, and the male orgasm will be optimum! And because many men can't stand the missionary position, they may not be able to ejaculate when they're in it.

Attention, Ladies

After intercourse, do what you feel like doing: sleep, urinate, eat, walk. You *don't* need to do the "bicycle" for 15 minutes, or lie back with your knees up, or refrain from urinating. To avoid infection, it is wise to urinate immediately after intercourse.

However, many fertility experts report that in some instances, lying quietly in bed for 15–20 minutes after intercourse, can help the conception process.

Anejaculation

This refers to men who do not or cannot ejaculate when they climax. Sometimes anejaculation occurs only with intercourse and not masturbation; often the problem exists with both sexual acts. This is obviously a cause of infertility, but it is difficult to diagnose and depends on *self-reporting*. If your partner is well lubricated, she may not realize that you have this problem either. It's also important not to confuse anejaculation with *retrograde ejaculation*, where the ejaculate goes backward rather than forward, a true structural problem that can be diagnosed and treated (see chapters 4 and 6).

Anejaculation is a problem rooted in psychological trauma, and is an indication that you need counseling. If you suffer from this, you must report it to avoid long, involved workups. Either a primary care doctor or a urologist can refer you to a therapist who specializes in this problem.

A Word About Arousal

Getting yourself aroused when you're having sex by the calendar can be a challenge. Feel free to use as many visual aids as you like: videos, magazines, strip-teases, soft lights, and so on. Research indicates that when a woman reaches orgasm at the time of ejaculation (but not before), her orgasmic contractions also help to propel the sperm upward, toward the uterus. If a woman reaches orgasm prior to ejaculation (i.e., during foreplay), the contractions may keep sperm away. Try to time your orgasms if you can. You should also avoid alcohol, marijuana, cocaine, and all the other no-no's mentioned in the "Bad Habits" section. You should probably avoid flavored sex jellies or other lubricant concoctions, since they may interfere with sperm quality or cervical mucus. Vibrators and dildos are fine as long as they're clean! Finally, avoid intercourse in the shower, pool, hot tub, whirlpool or bathtub; water may interfere with either sperm quality or cervical mucus; heat will interfere with sperm production.

7. Work Habits

In the "Coping Habits" section, I touched on the issue of work-related stress, which can interfere with ovulation as well as reduce sperm count. Job stress is caused either by working too many hours or by having to perform well under rigid scrutiny (this scrutiny is often self-imposed). But often these two conditions are combined, creating impossible schedules and goal setting for the worker, spawning a new addiction known as "workaholism," discussed below.

The physical position (i.e., sitting all day) you maintain as you perform your job function can also affect fertility, while the level of toxins you're exposed to in the workplace is a major factor in reducing both male and female fertility. These issues are discussed separately in the "Occupational Hazards" section.

Workaholism

You are considered a workaholic when your job takes priority over your personal life or when you spend more time at your work than you do at home. The term *workaholic* has unfortunately come to have *positive* connotations in our society. Many companies and firms pride themselves on employing workaholics, devaluing employees who want to work reasonable hours. As a result, a new term, *work addiction* has come to replace *workaholism*. People who are self-employed or who run businesses are also classic workaholics.

We now know that there is a real *physical* addiction that workaholics experience, as well as common personality traits. (Being called a "Type A" personality is used interchangeably with the term *workaholic*.) Workaholics tend to be overachievers, often setting goals that are so high they are unreachable. Working to reach the goal sets off a complex chain of adrenaline rushes that feed the work addiction. The workaholic actually gets high on that adrenaline rush and misses the rush when he or she is not at work. This is why workaholics prefer to spend their weekends at work rather than home, and typically work a 5–9 schedule rather than 9–5.

Many people hide from personal problems by overworking. In fact, personal stress can often *trigger* a work addiction. This is particularly common when couples experience a delay in conception. To avoid dealing with possible infertility, one or both partners will often become "too busy" to really try, using their "impossible" schedules as a cover for a real physical problem. Women who have infertile male partners will often become work "widows" as the male partners develop work addictions to avoid going home and facing their feelings of inadequacy. This issue is addressed more in chapters 4 and 6.

Whether you use the office as a refuge or you thrive on the rush of overachieving, the lack of quality time at home will affect your desire for sex as well as your reproductive capacity. In addition, work addiction will often foster other bad habits: poor nutrition, smoking, drinking, overexercising, and so on. The group *Workaholics Anonymous*, listed in your local White Pages, is a 12-step program designed to help work addicts lead healthier, personal lives. Your primary care physician can also refer you to a counselor or therapist who can help you break your addiction.

Occupational Hazards

While there are numerous things we can do to purify our bodies and our food intake, many of us face daily toxins in our workplace that can affect our fertility.

Of the roughly 60,000 industrial chemicals used, only three have been documented as absolutely affecting human reproduction: metallic lead (still found in many gasolines and exhausts), the pesticide dibromochloropropane (DCBP), and a pharmaceutical solvent called ethylene oxide. Several other chemicals have been linked to impaired fertility, causing either reduced sperm counts or ovarian failure. These chemicals include mercury, chlordecone (another pesticide), vinyl chloride (do you work in a hard-plastics plant?), a variety of paints, solvents, stains, and varnishes, and manganese (used in steel, glass, ink, ceramics, paints, welding rods, rubber, and wood preservatives). Some of the industries where harmful chemicals are commonplace are agriculture, laboratories, oil, chemical and atomic industries, pulp and paper, and textiles.

New evidence suggests that several chemicals break down into an "estrogenic" by-product. In other words, many chemicals actually "leak" a substance identical to the female hormone estrogen. This is being linked to reduced sperm counts, a rise in male anatomical problems such as undescended testes, and a rise in certain reproductive cancers, including breast cancer.

The list of damaging toxins is dizzying, overwhelming, and upsetting. The best thing you can do is inform yourself about your workplace hazards by consulting the appropriate departments within the Environmental Protection Agency (EPA) in the United States or within Environment Canada. You can also go directly to the industry in question (such as the Department of Agriculture). Environmental groups such as Greenpeace have information on a number of industry hazards. In the meantime, you can review Tables 1, 2, and 3 for more information. These tables list suspected occupational hazards as of 1982.

Ladies only

If you work in a dental office as a dentist, dental hygienist, or dental assistant, it's now known that nitrous oxide can dramatically affect your ability to either conceive or sustain a pregnancy. Although nitrous oxide is also used in veterinary clinics, ambulances, and hospitals, dental office workers are exposed to higher levels because no masks are placed on patients' mouths. If you're exposed to five or more hours of "unscavenged" (unmasked) nitrous oxide, your fertility can be dramatically compromised. One study found that women exposed to these amounts experienced a 60% drop in conception rates with each menstrual cycle, while 50% of the pregnant women in the study exposed to these levels miscarried.

As for the hazards of video display terminals (VDTs), this scare was most prevalent in the early 1980s when miscarriage rates seemed to increase among VDT users. There is not yet any conclusive link between VDTs and miscarriages, but all women can now get screens to place over their VDTs to filter out any suspect radiation.

Occupational hazards you can do something about

One of the chief occupational workplace hazards is being exposed to secondhand smoke. No one in 1995 should put up with this. Many workplaces are now smoke free, but there are a disturbing number of companies that are not smoke-free working, or do not enforce smoke-free policies. Most states and provinces now have rigid legislation regarding smoking in the workplace. You can arrange to have an occupational health and/or safety representative inspect your workplace and fine your employer if the company isn't complying with state or provincial laws. Most of these agencies accept anonymous complaints so your job is not compromised. In most states and provinces, employers have a legal responsibility to provide a clean workplace; if you feel you must leave your workplace because of secondhand smoke, you are in a good position to sue your employer.

Similarly, long hours of overtime work must be compensated with either equal time off or overtime pay. You should not be expected to endure repeated episodes of double shifts or twelve-hour days without compensation.

If you're in a sedentary job where you sit for long periods of time, schedule time out for stretching and walking around. Again, males may be prone to reduced sperm production due to raising the temperature of their testes (see the "Personal Hygiene" section above).

Finally, anyone who works around radiation, such as healthcare professionals and technicians, should arrange to wear a shield over his or her pelvic region to protect the reproductive organs.

As I stated at the beginning of this chapter, it's crucial to assess whether your lifestyle habits are posing any hazards to your fertility. If you and your partner are trying to conceive, you should clean up your act in terms of bad habits, exercise, and nutrition *before* you begin charting the menstrual cycle and timing intercourse. Otherwise, you could be wasting a lot of time and energy—something an infertility investigation is dependent on. The next chapter is the next step in the fertility journey. Understanding your individual ovulation cycle as a *couple* is a must if you're trying to conceive.

Table 1: Some Chemical Hazards That May Affect Reproductive Health

Hazard	Workers at Risk	Potential Reproductive Effect	Protective Measures
Anesthetic Gases (including halothane, nitrous oxide, methoxyflurane)	health care workers in hospitals and dental clinics, veterinary surgeons and assistants, researchers in animal laboratories	male workers: sperm abnormalities; wives/female partners of exposed male workers may experience an increased evidence of miscarriages, premature deliveries, and offspring with birth defects; female workers: same as wives/female partners of male workers; the fetus: birth defects	install scavenger units to collect stray gases; monitor air in operating theatre to ensure low levels
Benzene	workers producing or using solvents, plastics, rubbers, glues, dyes, detergents, paints, petroleum, and other products containing this substance	male and female workers: chromosome changes, linked with leukemia and genetic effects in offspring; female workers: prolonged menstrual bleeding and postpartum hemmorhage after chronic exposure; the fetus: birth defects, higher incidence of leukemia, illness from contaminated breast milk	substitute non toxic or less toxic products; take regular workplace air samples; ensure proper ventilation and safe engineering processes
Beryllium	ceramic makers, electronics workers, jewelry makers, laboratory workers, nuclear technologists	female workers: pregnancy may exacerbate symptoms of beryllium poisoning and cause death; the fetus: may cross placenta and affect fetal development	monitor workplace levels regularly; install proper ventilation and dust collection devices in the work environment
Carbon Disulfide	degreasers, glue makers, paint removers, rubber makers, rayon viscose makers	male workers: decreased libido, impotence, sperm abnormalities; female workers: irregular menstrual cycle, decreased fertility, frequent miscarriages; the fetus: higher incidence of miscarriage	monitor workplace levels and reduce to minimum; ensure that prolonged worker exposure is prohibited
Hormones (including androgens, estrogens, progestogens, and synthetic products such as DES)	workers involved in the extraction, manufacture, and use of hormones, including pharmaceutical workers, laboratory workers, farmers, and veterinarians	male workers: sexual impotence, breast enlargement, infertility; female workers: irregular menstruation, infertility, ovarian cysts, breast lumps, cancer of the reproductive system; the fetus: may develop enlarged breasts and other signs of sex-	monitor regularly to ensure low levels of airborne hormones; isolate the process through engineering design

Substance	Health Effects	Workers at Risk	Precautions
	ual maturity as well as abnormalities of the skeletal system, heart, and windpipe; DES may cause cancer in female offspring, genital and sperm abnormalities in male offspring		
Lead	male workers: decreased libido, decreased sperm count, atrophy of the testes; wives/female partners demonstrate adverse effects such as infertility, menstrual disorders, miscarriages; female workers: infertility, miscarriages, stillbirths, menstrual disorders; the fetus: higher incidence of miscarriages, stillbirths, neonatal death; mental retardation can occur; newborns can be affected by contaminated breast milk	auto manufacturers, ceramic and pottery makers, electronics workers, farmers, pesticide makers, paint makers and users, and typographers	sample workplace air frequently; provide adequate ventilation; clean work areas regularly
Mercury	male workers: reduced fertility; female workers: miscarriages, stillbirths; the fetus: linked with severe brain damage, mental retardation, increased rate of miscarriages and stillbirths	battery makers, ceramic workers, commercial fishermen, dental workers, farm workers, jewelry makers, lithographers, pesticide makers, photographic chemical makers and users	regular air monitoring and good ventilation; enclose mercury processes; check frequently for spills and vapor leaks
Pesticides (including carbaryl, dibromochloropropane, kepone, malathion 2,4,5-T)	male workers: chromosomal changes, impotence, loss of libido, decreased sperm counts, atrophy of the testes; female workers: miscarriages, chromosomal changes; the fetus: miscarriages, birth deformities	agricultural workers, commercial and household gardeners, pesticide manufacturers	design processes to prevent worker contact with substance; monitor air levels in workplace and keep to a minimum
Vinyl Chloride	male workers: genetic damage of the sperm, leading to adverse pregnancy outcome in wives/female partners; female workers: genetic damage to ovum, miscarriages, stillbirths; the fetus: higher incidence of miscarriage, fetal death and birth defects; may develop cancer after exposure during pregnancy	workers involved in the production of vinyl chloride and polyvinyl chloride and its related products	monitor workplace regularly; use proper ventilation and safe design to keep levels at a minimum

Source: *The Canadian Advisory Council on the Status of Women, Ottawa, 1982.*

Table 2: Some Biological Hazards That May Affect Reproductive Health

Hazard	Workers at Risk	Potential Reproductive Effect	Protective Measures
Brucellosis (Undulant fever)	animal breeders, farmers, health care workers, meat handlers, veterinarians	male and female workers: brueallae may lodge in reproductive organs, leading to local inflammations and infertility; the fetus: miscarriage, developmental defects	control infection in animals; use caution in handling diseased animals and their products as well as the urine and feces of infected humans
Chicken Pox (Varicella)	day care workers, pediatric nurses, teachers, laboratory workers, parents	the fetus: prematurity, retardation, muscular, skeletal, and heart defects, increased incidence of neonatal death	isolate infectious person and handle contaminated articles using aseptic techniques; pregnant women should avoid exposure
Cytomegalovirus	blood bank workers, health care workers, dental workers, laboratory workers	the fetus: infection leading to jaundice, enlarged spleen and liver, heart, eye, and central nervous system damage in the newborn	use care in handling sputum, urine, semen, blood, and other secretions of the human body; pregnant women should avoid exposure
Hepatitis (Infectious and Serum)	blood unit workers, kidney dialysis technicians, laundry workers, laboratory workers, sterilization unit workers	the fetus: infection leading to miscarriage, prematurity, stillbirth, and jaundice; enlarged spleen, increased death rate in newborns	isolate infectious individuals; label potentially infectious specimens visibly; use disposable needles, syringes, lancets where possible; pregnant women should avoid exposure
Herpes Virus Hominus	health care workers, hospital staff, laboratory workers, research scientists	male and female workers: transmissible genital infections; the fetus: fetal death, miscarriage, liver and eye diseases, central nervous system damage	isolate infected persons or specimens; use caution in handling infected objects

Disease	Workers at Risk	Effects	Precautions
Mumps (Infectious Parotitis)	childcare workers, hospital staff, laboratory workers, restaurant workers, teachers, parents	male and female workers: inflammation of testes and ovaries, leading to infertility or sterility; the fetus: miscarriages, stillbirths, developmental defects, hydrocephalus	isolate infectious persons, handle specimens with care; alert all workers potentially in contact; promote immunization
Rubella (German Measles)	childcare workers, hospital personnel, laboratory staff, restaurant workers, teachers, parents	the fetus: placental infection may lead to severe congenital abnormalities including deafness, blindness, heart defects, mental retardation	promote immunization; isolate infected person; handle contaminated material with care; pregnant women must avoid exposure
Syphilis	blood unit workers, health care workers, laboratory workers	male and female workers: secondary lesions in organs of the body including reproductive organs, infertility or sterility; the fetus: embryal death, infection leading to liver and spleen enlargement, developmental defects	avoid contact with infected lesions; exercise caution in handling infected equipment
Tuberculosis	dairy farm workers, health care workers, laboratory workers, laundry workers	male and female workers: tubercular infection of the reproductive organs; the fetus: can be infected through blood transfer from the mother or by aspiration of amniotic fluid	promote immunization; test animals regularly; handle infected specimens with caution

Source: The Canadian Advisory Council on the Status of Women, Ottawa, 1982.

Table 3: Some Physical Hazards That May Affect Reproductive Health

Hazard	Workers at Risk	Potential Reproductive Effect	Protective Measures
Ionizing Radiation	atomic radiation workers, dental and chiropractor office workers, hospital employees, scientists	male and female workers: sterility, premature aging of the sex cells, altered genetic material; the fetus: damage resulting in prenatal death, mental retardation, birth defects, increased incidence of leukemia and other cancers	reduce workplace levels to a minimum; use proper shielding techniques; monitor individual exposures using filmbadge dosimeters and other mobile measuring devices; leave contaminated workclothes at the worksite; maintain exposure records for workers
Noise and Vibration	assembly line workers, airline attendants, construction workers, garment and textile workers, machinists, motor vehicle drivers, pneumatic drill operators	male workers: sexual dysfunction and decreased fertility; female workers: disturbances of the menstrual cycle, increased rate of premature births and complications during labor; the fetus: disturbances of uterine circulation in the mother may lead to miscarriage, low birth weight, perinatal mortality	design machines to ensure minimal noise and vibration; use proper preventive maintenance for equipment; isolate noise using noise absorbing partitions; use sound and sound and vibration absorbing material in floors, walls, and ceilings; install mufflers on all motorized equipment, provide frequent rest periods and job rotations to decrease worker exposure
Non-ionizing Radiation	flight attendants and pilots, food service workers, health care workers, radio navigation and radar communication workers	male workers: degeneration of the testes, decreased libido, lower sperm count and motility, abnormally shaped sperm; female workers: changes in menstrual cycles, decreased lactation in nursing mothers; the fetus: miscarriage, retarded fetal development, congenital defects such as club foot and Down's syndrome	shield or isolate operations using non-ionizing radiation; check sources regularly for production of X-rays
Temperature (Heat)	workers in bakeries, canneries, foundries, garment and textile factories, laundries, mines, smelters	male workers: decreased sperm count, atrophy of the testes; female workers: decreased fertility; the fetus: increased embryal death, low birth weight	provide adequate training and acclimation, properly designed clothing, and frequent rest periods; enclose heat producing operations as much as possible; ventilate the work area

Source: The Canadian Advisory Council on the Status of Women, Ottawa, 1982.

3

Zen and the Art of
Menstrual Cycle Maintenance

When it comes to understanding the female menstrual cycle, there *is* a great deal of Zen involved. In a word, Zen boils down to *acceptance*. Most women of reproductive age today haven't learned to accept the timing of their natural cycles because many of them have been trained to medicate them in an attempt to alleviate the uncomfortable premenstrual symptoms that precede or accompany their periods. Often, women will be put on oral contraceptives in their teens and twenties, not as a form of birth control, but as a way of altering the cycle to make it more regular or bearable. Many of these women will simply stay on oral contraceptives (OCs) until they want to conceive. In extreme cases, some women who suffer from premenstrual syndrome (PMS) are put on a hormonal therapy, which may include danazol. Danazol actually *shuts down* ovarian function, mimicking menopause. And there are published case studies in which some women have been recommended for a hysterectomy as a way to treat PMS.

The bottom line is that many women planning to conceive have no idea what kind of menstrual cycle they have because the cycle has been masked for so long. This means that most couples need to formaly introduce themselves to the female menstrual cycle. This chapter is designed to tell you everything you need to know about the female menstrual cycle to plan conception. Obviously, much of the information in this chapter will be better understood by women than men. However, I have included a special section at the end of the chapter for men. Observing the menstrual cycle can be a challenging task, and there is a role the male can play in the charting process. The male hormonal cycle is discussed in chapter 4.

An Unremarkable Menstrual Cycle

Remember that lecture in health class, when the teacher warned all the girls that they could get pregnant at *any* time—during their periods, after their periods, and so on? *Well, it's not true.* Young women are told this because it's assumed that most teens are *not* aware of their menstrual cycles. In addition, because many teenage women have *irregular* menstrual cycles (extremely common from the time of *menarche*, the first period, until about age 18 or 19), practicing natural birth control isn't a practical option for them. So, for a sexually active 17-year-old, warning her that she "can get pregnant during her period" is still a good idea.

Once you reach your mid-to-late 20s, your natural menstrual cycle will probably have established itself and will become fairly regular. But what's regular for one person may be irregular for someone else.

Your menstrual cycle is actuall a "hormonal cycle." It's driven by a symphony of hormones that trigger one another, stopping and starting, flooding and tapering in a regular rhythm each month. Every woman's hormones dance to a different tune, but rarely does this pattern correspond to the English calendar. This is because the word *month* comes from the root word *moon*. The Greek word for moon is *mene*, and *menstruation* actually means "moon-change." This is why some women have shorter and longer cycles. In fact, female roommates who have completely different cycles in the beginning may synchronize their cycles over time. Some experts suggest that women may produce pheromones (a sexual odor) that other women can unconsciously smell. At any rate, women's cycles are often more "in tune" with the moon and with each other, on levels not completely understood.

The Hormonal Cycle

Every woman is born with about 400,000 million potential eggs in her ovaries. That number dwindles throughout her childhood and over the 30-odd years that she menstruates. Any eggs that remain dissolve into the ovarian tissue, and at this point the woman officially enters menopause. Low levels of sex hormones are continuously produced during a woman's reproductive years. But it is the continuous *fluctuation* of hormones that establish the menstrual cycle and the understandable premenstrual symptoms.

The main organs involved in the cycle are the hypothalamus (a part of the brain), the pituitary gland, and the ovaries. The hypothalamus is like the symphony conductor, controlling and signaling each hormonal "instrument" to do its solo, duet, and so on. It tells the pituitary gland to start the hormonal "program", which signals the ovaries to begin their performance by producing estrogen and progesterone. The hypothalamus is sensitive to the fluctuating levels of hormones produced by the ovaries. When the level of estrogen drops below a certain level, the hypothalamus turns on gonadotropin-releasing hormone *(GnRH)*, which stimulates the pituitary gland to release follicle stimulating hormone *(FSH)*. FSH triggers the growth of 10–20 ovarian follicles, but only one of them will mature fully; the others will start to degenerate some time before ovulation. As the follicles grow, they secrete estrogen in increasing amounts. The estrogen affects the lining of the uterus, signaling it to enter the proliferatory, or growth, phase. When the egg approaches maturity inside the mature follicle, the follicle releases a burst of progesterone (progesterone is also referred to as the propregnancy hormone) in addition to the estrogen. This progesterone/estrogen combination triggers the hypothalamus to release more GnRH, which signals the pituitary gland to secrete FSH and luteinizing hormone *(LH)*. When FSH and LH levels peak—known as the *LH surge*—this signals the follicle to release the egg, resulting in ovulation. Home test kits are now on the market that will detect the LH surge in your cycle.

Under the influence of LH, the follicle changes its function and becomes a *corpus luteum* (meaning "yellow body" because it actually *turns* yellow), secreting decreasing amounts of estrogen and increasing amounts of progesterone. The progesterone influences the estrogen-primed uterine lining to secrete fluids that nourish the egg (the secretory phase). Immediately after ovulation, FSH returns to normal, or base levels, and the LH decreases gradually as the progesterone increases. If the egg is fertilized, the corpus luteum continues to secrete estrogen and progesterone to maintain the pregnancy. The corpus luteum is stimulated by human chorionic gonadotropin (HCG), a hormone secreted by the developing placenta. (HCG secretion is what a home pregnancy test detects in the urine.) If the egg isn't fertilized, the corpus luteum degenerates until it becomes nonfunctioning, at which point it is called a *corpus albicans*. As degeneration progresses, progesterone levels decrease. The decreased progesterone fails to maintain the uterine lining, which causes it to shed. The shedding of the lining is menstruation. All the cramps that may accompany your period are caused by uterine contractions, which help squeeze the lining out. Then, the whole cycle starts again.

To simplify this, imagine listening to Beethoven's Fifth Symphony. It begins with "G-n-R-H. G-n-R-H." The next octave starts with "F-S-H-F-S-H-F-S-H-F-S-H," which continues until the symphony changes again, this time with "LH." As you hear bursts from some instruments and longer solos from others, imagine estrogen and progesterone pulsing and bursting into the bloodstream in precise, controlled amounts. When the symphony is over, the woman menstruates.

Female Ovulation Cycle

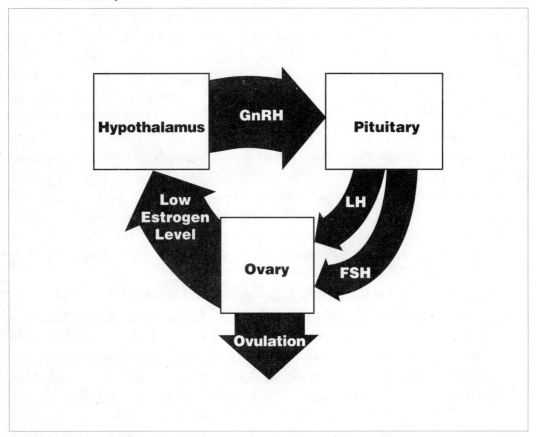

Figure 1.
Reprinted with permission of Serono Canada, Inc., 1994.

Then the symphony starts over again. As we all know, however, each conductor has a different *interpretation* of a piece of music. Some use more strings, while others use more horns; some quicken the pace of the music, while others slow it down. All women's hormonal cycles play the same piece of music, but the rhythms, timing, and pace of that music will vary from conductor to conductor. (The cycle is illustrated in Figure 1.)

The first period, called *menarche*, usually starts in the middle of puberty, at around 12 or 13 years of age. The first few periods are sporadic, and it's not uncommon for periods to be irregular for a couple of years. Periods continue until about 48 or 49 years of age, and then start to get sporadic again, tapering off as menopause sets in. Few cycles are actually 28 days. Where does the number 28 come from? The figure is only an average representing the cycle length of thousands of women added together and divided by the number of women. It is therefore a *statistical* average, not a figure that refers to the typical number of days in a woman's cycle. Menstrual cycles range anywhere from 20 to 40 days, and the bleeding lasts anywhere from 2–8 days, 4–6 days being the average.

There's a big difference between your own cycle and a calendar month, however. Because your cycle length may be shorter or longer than the 30- or 31-day calendar month, the calendar date of your period may vary from month to month. That's why it's a good idea to keep a written record of your period. (Charting is discussed further below.) Each month has a different number of days, so unless you were consistently irregular, you couldn't menstruate on exactly the 15th of each month.

It's important to count *the first day of bleeding as day one of your cycle*. Although many women count the first day of clear discharge *after* their periods as day one, this is not as accurate. What's the difference? Because ovulation always takes place roughly 14 days before your next period, five days off in your counting could radically interfere with your family planning. When you're on OCs, the first day of bleeding is *always* counted as day one. So, when you go off the OCs, your cycle is more accurately tracked by using the same counting method. Also, doctors always count the first day of bleeding as day one of the cycle, and it's crucial to accurately establish the date of your last menstrual period prior to conception when your pregnant.

By the way, many women assume that their menstrual flow is made up of only blood, but this is not so. The menstrual fluid consists of a variety of ingredients: cervical and vaginal mucus, degenerated endometrial particles, and blood. The fluid does not smell until it makes contact with bacteria in the air and starts to decompose.

Irregular Cycles

One of the most common fertility problems is an irregular menstrual cycle. But before you jump to the conclusion that you're irregular, it's important to remember that being regular doesn't mean your cycle is the same number of days each time. One month your cycle may be 29 days, and the next month it may be 31 days. This is still considered the norm. It's also normal to be lighter one month and heavier the next. As long as you're menstruating every 20–40 days, it's a sign that you're ovulating. Another common misconception about irregular cycles is that unless you have a period every four weeks (again, the statistical average) you're irregular. This is not true. Some women menstruate every three weeks; some menstruate every five weeks. The only times you should be concerned is if your period consistently yo-yos: three weeks, then four weeks, then five weeks, then three weeks, and so forth. When this happens, it's usually a sign that you're not ovulating regularly. This is common in young girls after they first begin menstruating, but it is not normal in women who are in their mid-20s or older. If your period jumps around once or twice a year, you don't have anything to worry about. Occasional stress is usually the culprit when this happens. However, poor nutrition, overexercising, and indulging in some of the lifestyle vices discussed in chapter 2 can cause a menstrual cycle to yo-yo.

When you've skipped a period

Obviously, skipping a period when you're trying to conceive may be due to pregnancy. But women may skip a period from time to time and then experience a heavier flow with their next period. This is extremely common. Women who are trying to get pregnant, however, often fear that this is a mild miscarriage—so mild that it simply feels like a heavy period. This usually is not the case. Although it's possible for a pregnancy not to take and expel in the menstrual flow, it's rare and occurs in less than 1% of women. If it were to occur, it would be so early a pregnancy that the term *miscarriage* would be totally inappropriate; it would simply be a pregnancy that wasn't yet established, technically called a "blighted ovum." Skipping one period in most cases is caused by stress. The flow is heavier after a skipped period because the estrogen has been building up in the endometrium longer, and there is more lining than usual that needs to be shed. In essence, you would have built up two cycles' worth of lining, so the flow is naturally heavier than normal.

It's also common to skip a period altogether and *not* experience a heavier flow the next time around. This means you actually skipped an *ovulation* cycle and had not produced a lining in your endometrium that would support a pregnancy. In this case, there wasn't a lining to shed.

Causes of irregular or missed cycles

The number-one cause of a skipped period is pregnancy. Other causes of irregular or skipped periods are emotional stress or what I call "nutritional abuse." These problems are discussed in detail in chapter 2.

For some women, the cause of irregular cycles could be a thyroid disorder of some sort. The thyroid gland regulates your metabolism by secreting thyroid hormone. When the gland is overactive and secretes too much thyroid hormone, known as *hyperthyroidism*, you can either miss periods or have a much longer cycle than normal, and your period is shorter, with a scanty or light flow. On the flip side, when the gland is underactive and doesn't secrete *enough* hormone, known as *hypothyroidism*, your cycles can become shorter, while the period itself is longer with a much heavier flow than normal. Thyroid problems occur in about one in twenty people worldwide but affect women about seven times as often. If this is the cause of your menstrual irregularity, it is easily remedied. Once your thyroid problem is treated, your periods will simply return to normal.

Finally, irregular cycles may be normal for your *age*. For example, it often takes young women several years before they establish a regular menstrual cycle, which is why many young women will be put on oral contraceptives to regulate their periods. Women beyond 40 could begin menopause at any time, and irregular cycles may be a sign of perimenopause, which is addressed in chapters 5 and 6.

Amenorrhea: No Menstrual Cycle

There *is* such a thing as having no menstrual cycle; however, if you don't begin menstruating by the age of 18, you probably have a hormonal imbalance that can be easily remedied with hormonal supplements. If you're menstruating regularly and are between 20 and 40 years of age, it's unusual to simply stop menstruating. If this does occur, nutritional abuse is the most common cause. When the female body is malnourished, it stops ovulating because it can't sustain a pregnancy. (See chapter 2 for more details.) Athletes in intensive training may also experience amenorrhea.

Amenorrhea can be caused by either an overactive or underactive thyroid gland. If this is the case, once your thyroid problem is treated, you should begin menstruating again. In all other cases of a stopped or stunted menstrual cycle, progesterone supplements will remedy it.

Why you need to bleed

Today, because there are fewer pregnancies and a longer life cycle, women have to deal with more periods in their lifetime than did women in the past. Also, in the past century women have experienced a radical change in their diet, environment, stress levels, career, and family expectations. Understandably, the combination of all these factors has affected the hormonal cycle of women, which, in turn, impacts the menstrual cycle.

Again, it's fine to skip a period once in a while or experience some occasional fluctuation. But if you've missed more than two periods and know for certain that you're not pregnant (confirmed by either a pregnancy test or the absence of any sexual activity), then you need to see your doctor and have your period "induced." You'll simply be given a progesterone supplement, which will kick-start your cycle again. It's dangerous to go longer than three months without a "bleed." If the uterus isn't regularly "cleaned out," you can be at risk of developing uterine cancer.

When You Have a Heavy Flow (Menorrhagia)

If you have an extremely heavy flow, it may be normal for you. This is known as *primary menorrhagia*, which means that your flow has been heavy since you first began menstruating. If this is the case, there isn't anything to worry about. You should have your blood levels checked about every six months, however, because a consistent heavy flow is the number-one cause of anemia.

If a light flow slowly *develops* into a heavy flow, this is known as *secondary menorrhagia*. When this happens, as long as you're having annual pelvic exams and biannual blood tests, you shouldn't be concerned. If your flow *suddenly* becomes unexplainably heavy, see your doctor. This kind of menorrhagia may signify other problems such as fibroids or tumors. Flows are considered dangerously heavy if you need to change your pad or tampon every hour.

When You Have Painful Periods (Dysmenorrhea)

Primary dysmenorrhea means that you've had painful periods ever since you started menstruating. *Secondary dysmenorrhea* involves periods that have become more painful over time. In either case, painful periods are common, and there are medications that can alleviate cramps. Cramps are simply caused by uterine contractions, which pushes out the lining; some uteri contract more than others. Taking an anti-inflammatory medication such as *naproxen sodium* (Anaprox), for example, *before* your period starts, can help. (Younger women will often be placed on OCs to help alleviate painful periods.) It's also important to judge normal cramping from unusual, debilitating pain during your periods. Endometriosis, a serious disease, is often the culprit behind severe pain during your period. When your pain keeps you from participating in pleasurable activities, there's about a 40% chance that your pain is caused by endometriosis. (See chapter 6 for more information).

If You've Been on Oral Contraceptives

It's common for younger women, in particular, to be placed on OCs as a way of controlling severe PMS symptoms, irregular cycles, or dysmenorrhea. When you're on OCs periods are a dream come true. Cramps are relatively mild, flow is medium to light, and the periods are punctual to the point where you can set your watch by them. However, many women are surprised to find that when they go *off* OCs, their menstrual problems return. If their cycles were irregular before the oral contraceptives, they will continue to be irregular after they go off them; if they suffered from painful periods before, they probably will have painful periods after. Oral contraceptives are only a temporary panacea for menstrual cycle problems.

Some women will remain regular when they go off oral contraceptives, though. This is usually because when they initially went on them, they were younger and had less mature ovulation cycles. *Ovulation cycles mature as you get into your 20s and 30s, which is why the cycles will normalize.* But often the original cycle, however flawed, returns. Furthermore, it can take up to *six months* for your ovulation cycle to kick in and return to normal. When you're planning to conceive, allow at least that much time. Doctors will advise you to wait until you get two natural periods before you try to conceive. This is fine, but don't panic if you don't conceive after your third, fourth, or fifth cycle. There is a delusion that as soon as we go off oral contraceptives we'll get pregnant. This is just not true. Perfectly fertile couples having intercourse every other day can wait a year before conception actually takes place.

Fertility Awareness 101

Fertility awareness techniques, which have been around since antiquity, gained popularity in the 1970s so women could practice natural birth control. By the 1980s, these same techniques were used for the opposite purpose: to plan conception. Yet, in the 1990s no woman outside of a monogamous, HIV-negative relationship has the luxury of practicing natural birth control because of the risk of being exposed to sexually transmitted diseases (STDs). So, unfortunately, learning to read the menstrual cycle has become a lost art. In fact, most women are menstrually "illiterate" until they decide to have a child.

As discussed above, few menstrual cycles are an exact number of days each month. Some women may have a 33-day cycle one month, a 36-day cycle the next, and a 31-day cycle the next. In my own case, I have cycles that run anywhere between 35 and 45 days, and I *never* know how many days to expect between cycles. And I am *not* an unusual "menstrual cycle statistic" by any means. Cycles like these create problems for women trying to conceive, because there is a very small time frame within our cycle when we actually *can* conceive.

We are fertile during ovulation, which takes place about 14 days before our *next* period begins. Women with predictable menstrual cycles can easily use a calendar to "catch" the fertile peak in their cycles. For example, a woman with an average 28-day cycle would circle day 14 of the cycle on her calendar and begin having frequent intercourse between day 12 and day 16. Women with unpredictable or irregular cycles will have a much harder time doing this. Fortunately, there are several fertility awareness techniques for women who are not born "calendar girls." You'll get the best results if you combine *all* of these methods together!

Charting Your Menstrual Cycle

There's no way of knowing how regular your cycles are until you start to actually chart them. A classic case for charting exists when women decide to conceive after being on hormonal contraception for years.

For other women planning to conceive, charting serves some useful purposes. First, by charting your cycle, you'll become aware of your body's premenstrual symptoms, which are useful "precursors" to your period and hence, signs of when your fertile stage has begun or *passed*. For instance, if you suffer from tender breasts roughly a week *before* your period, you might begin to notice a pattern of premenstrual breast pain that can *assist* you in establishing a pattern of fertility. Symptoms such as mood swings or bloating can be used in this way as well.

Second, charting your cycle will alert you to the problem of an irregular cycle, which could mean that you're ovulating irregularly or not at all. Correcting the underlying problem that's causing your irregular cycles may prevent delayed conception and save you needless frustration. Charting should be done for at least four cycles before an accurate pattern can be established.

A PMS *refresher*

Premenstrual syndrome (PMS), which has recently been revised in the psychiatric literature to *premenstrual dysphoric disorder* ("unhappy before your period"), is a real medical condition that affects about 40% of all women in their childbearing years. But because of the media circus that's made PMS famous, women have been bombarded with misinformation about the condition.

PMS is an extremely vague label. Because virtually all women experience some kind of premenstrual symptom (bloating, tender breasts, etc.) women who have *true* PMS have been lumped together with women who experience premenstrual symptoms that don't bother them all that much or affect their ability to function on a daily basis. In fact, 90% of women who menstruate experience premenstrual symptoms of some sort. It's all part of the normal, hormonal changes that are occurring. Yet 10% of menstruating women experience no symptoms before their period.

Of the 90% who do experience PMS, half will experience the more traditional symptoms such as breast tenderness, bloating, food cravings, irritability, and mood swings. For many women, these symptoms are welcomed because they indicate that all is well and alert them that their period is on the way. These symptoms are the natural, outward signs for the remarkable fluctuations in hormone levels that a woman undergoes every month when she menstruates (or even after a hysterectomy if her ovaries are still in place).

Out of the remaining 45% of women who experience premenstrual symptoms, 35–40% suffer the same symptoms of the first group, but in a more severe form. Their breasts are so sensitive that they hurt when lightly touched. They have severe bloating to the extent that they gain about five pounds before their periods. Instead of just food cravings, they may suddenly find that they have voracious appetites; instead of just being irritable, they may find that they become impossible to be around. Believe it or not, even these more severe symptoms are considered very normal.

The remaining 5–10% of women who experience premenstrual symptoms suffer from incapacitating symptoms, the kind the media has overreported. So it's perhaps more accurate to say that out of the 90% of women who experience some form of PMS, 80% experience premenstrual *symptoms*, and only 10% suffer from an actual premenstrual *syndrome* that has a real, negative affect on their lifestyle.

When doctors refer to *true* PMS, they are referring to both the severe premenstrual *symptom* group and the group that is incapacitated by their symptoms to the point where it is a true *syndrome*. PMS is a kind of umbrella term that refers to a cluster of physical and emotional symptoms that occur 1 to 14 days before the period that significantly interfere with a woman's interpersonal relationships and daily activities, and that disappear at or during menstruation. The symptoms are diverse and affect almost every part of the body. The following list of physical symptoms is only a sample of what some women report: breast swelling and tenderness, weight gain and abdominal bloating, constipation or diarrhea, headaches, acne or other skin eruptions, eye problems, joint and muscle pain, backache, sugar and salt cravings, increased appetite, fatigue, hoarseness, heart pounding, clumsiness and poor coordination, nausea, menopausallike hot sweats and chills, shakiness, dizziness, changes in sex drive (either more or less) sensitivity to noise, restlessness, insomnia, and even asthma and seizures.

The *emotional* symptoms of PMS often cause the most problems. They include sudden mood swings, melancholy, anxiety, irritability, emotional overresponsiveness, anger, rage, loss of control, depression, suicidal thoughts, nightmares, forgetfulness, confusion, decreased concentration, withdrawal, unexplained crying, inward anger, and physical or verbal aggression toward others.

Some women report increased energy levels, increased sexual drive, and bursts of creativity during this time. Even increased levels of anger and aggression can be viewed as constructive, particularly in business. Rents and bad debts are often collected at these times, and many women report that they are more productive in their work.

Using PMS to your advantage

If you menstruate chances are you experience some of the physical and emotional premenstrual symptoms. Through charting, you'll become more aware of your body and emotions at various stages in the menstrual cycle. Charting your symptoms is the only way doctors can actually *diagnose* PMS, since there isn't any blood test or diagnostic tool that can confirm the condition.

The idea is to use your own individual PMS symptoms as a marker for certain times in your cycle. For instance, when I get bloated and tender breasts around my period, it tends to occur about two weeks before my period, but *after* I've ovulated. Other women may notice tender breasts prior to or immediately after ovulation. It all depends on the individual. When I get weepy and irritable, my period is only a couple of days away, instead of a week away; other women may get weepy a week after ovulation, and so on.

How to create a symptom chart

On a separate daytimer, write down how you feel every day for three or four months. The chart should begin on day one of your cycle, which is when you actually start your bleed. Invent your own system for charting your symptoms. For example, you may want to separate your physical symptoms from your emotional symptoms and designate a number ranging from 1–10 (1 being less severe) to chart the intensity of your symptoms. You should also note any unusual activities that might increase your stress levels, such as getting laid off, moving, changing jobs, or fighting with a friend or family member. A sample follows.

If you compare the two charts, obviously you see more than just a change in numbers. The first chart looks as though some thought and logic went into it. In the second chart, everything—whether real or imagined—is exaggerated. The woman was even irritated by her own chart! So it's clear that the woman of January 17 is in a significantly worse mood than the woman of January 14. On the 14th, she was sincerely trying to be as accurate and scientific as possible; by the 17th, she was filling it out hastily, without as much care. Were her breasts really a 10 or were they in fact an 8.5? It doesn't matter. The second chart reveals a drastic change in her attitude and feelings—a strong indicator of how quickly her PMS symptoms overcame her and took hold of her lifestyle. Let's see how she feels after her period:

Cycle Day: 12   **Calendar Date: January 14/95**

Physical symptoms
Appetite = 5 (10 means voracious)
Cravings = 0 (10 means you have definite cravings)
Breasts = 3 (10 means they're really tender)
Bloat = 8 (10 means you're really bloated)
Weight = 3 pounds
Backache = 0 (10 means you're back is very achy)

Emotional symptoms
Mood = 4 (1 means happy; 10 means sad, depressed, etc.)
Irritability = 6 (1 means calm; 10 means really jumpy)
Energy = 7 (1 means low energy; 10 means high energy)
Sex drive = 7 (1 means low sex drive; 10 means high)
Stress = 6 (1 means low stress; 10 means high)

Special circumstances
—Got into an argument with Lee again. The usual. I feel fine. Just a little miffed.

Cycle Day: 15   **Calendar Date: January 17/95**

Physical symptoms
Appetite = 10
Cravings = 10 (chocolate)
Breasts = 10
Bloat = 10
Weight = 6 pounds (I'm a cow!)
Backache = 10

Emotional symptoms
Mood = 10!!!
Irritability = 10! 10! 10!
Energy = 0
Sex drive = 0
Stress = 10!

Special circumstances
—I hate my life!

Cycle Day: 5 (bleed—day 1 of the cycle—occurred on Jan. 30) Calendar Date: Feb. 4/95

Physical symptoms
Appetite = 3
Cravings = 0
Breasts = 0
Bloat = 0
Weight = normal
Backache = 0

Emotional symptoms
Mood = 1 (feeling really great!)
Irritability = 0
Energy = 10 (I actually did the laundry!)
Sex drive = 8
Stress = 1

Special circumstances
—Read my earlier charts! Don't know what came over me a couple of weeks ago!

The woman of February 4 is far happier, less stressed, and optimistic. She even has the wherewithal to observe how different she was acting just 18 days ago, about 13 days before her period. (Indeed, not all women experience PMS *exactly* 14 days before their period. It can vary. Fourteen days is just a rough number used when discussing an average 28-day cycle.) A sample of a more clinical chart—the kind your doctor may have on hand—is featured in figure 2.

Observing Cervical Mucus

This is a crucial fertility awareness method that any woman can easily get in the habit of doing. It also has the benefit of convenience, unlike the basal body temperature (BBT) method discussed below. This method is sometimes called the Billings method. Australians Evelyn and John Billings developed a way of interpreting the *changing consistency* of vaginal discharge, which is influenced by the cervical mucus bathing the vaginal walls. There are groups that now provide instruction in this technique. The most widely known is Serena, established and supported by the Roman Catholic Church. This group teaches the method only to married or monogamous couples who are Catholic. The Justisse Group, based in Canada, has consultants across the country who train women in both the United States and Canada to use this method. See the appendix for more information.

DAILY SYMPTOM RECORD

START DATE

DAY OF CYCLE	1	2	3	4	5	6	7	8	9	10	11	12	13	14	15	16	17	18	19	20	21	22	23	24	25	26	27	28
BLEEDING																												
SYMPTOMS																												
Irritable																												
Fatigue																												
Inward anger																												
Moody																												
Depressed																												
Restless																												
Anxious																												
Insomnia																												
Lack of control																												
Swelling																												
Bloating																												
Breast tenderness																												
Bowels: const. (C) loose (L)																												
Appetite (↑,↓)																												
Sex drive (↑,↓)																												
Chills (C); Sweats (S)																												
Headaches																												
Crave sweets, salt																												
Feel unattractive																												
Guilt																												
Unreasonable behavior																												
Low self-image																												
Nausea																												
Menstrual cramps																												
LIFESTYLE IMPACT																												
Aggressive toward others																												
Wish to be alone																												
Neglect housework																												
Time off work																												
Distractable, disorganized																												
Clumsy																												
Uneasy about driving																												
Suicidal thoughts																												
Stayed at home																												
LIFE EVENTS																												
Negative experience																												
Positive experience																												
Social activities																												
Vigorous exercise																												
MEDICATIONS																												

Your doctor may ask you to keep a diary of symptoms and their severity by filling out a chart similar to this.

INSTRUCTIONS

1. Consider the first day of bleeding as DAY 1 of your menstrual cycle.
2. Record your symptoms each evening at about the same time.
3. BLEEDING: Indicate bleeding by shading the box; indicate spotting with an X.
4. Fill in the box corresponding to a symptom by indicating the degree of severity as follows:

   MILD: 1 (Noticeable but not troublesome)

   MODERATE: 2 (Interferes with normal activity)

   SEVERE: 3 (Temporarily incapacitating)
5. MEDICATIONS: List these and enter an X on bad days when you take them.

(Modified with permission from PRISM Calendar, by Reid and Maddocks)

Figure 2. Sample form used for charting PMS symptoms.

Reprinted with permission of Syntex, Inc., 1994.

All you need to do is observe your toilet paper about twice a day, when you wipe yourself before or after going to the bathroom. Or, you can simply insert a finger into your vagina to collect whatever discharge is present. After your period finishes (i.e., your flow stops), you'll notice several days of no vaginal discharge at all (your dry days). Your vagina will still be moist, however, as it always is. Then, your mucus days will begin. The discharge starts out sticky, then gradually becomes creamier, wet, and slippery. Finally, on your peak day, the discharge has the consistency of egg white (some women describe it as snotlike), and will drip out of your vagina, evident when you wipe yourself or take off your underwear. This discharge will also be thinner, transparent, and stretchy, and you should be able to stretch it between two fingers. *This* mucus is your fertility marker. You will be ovulating either just *before* or just *after* it appears. This mucus will last for just about two days, then it will begin to get thicker and stickier. These are your postpeak days, also known as your luteal phase. This is when PMS symptoms will begin to make an appearance. The mucus will remain on the thicker, sticky side until your period starts. Then, the whole phase begins again.

To catch the peak, you'll need to begin having frequent intercourse (every other day) as your mucus days begin, and continue frequent intercourse until your postpeak mucus appears. Mucus usually develops between 3 and 9 days prior to ovulation. So you will probably need to have frequent intercourse for about two weeks. *Warning: This method is useless if you have a vaginal infection or untreated STD.*

You should also note your mucus observations on your symptom chart. Eventually, you should be able to link various premenstrual symptoms to a specific mucus consistency.

Guidelines for an accurate mucus chart

There are actually several steps involved in accurately observing your mucus. Since the chart depends on your observations throughout the day, record your observations before you go to bed at the end of the day. Never observe after intercourse, because you'll confuse semen and your sexual secretions with your own mucus. You should also refrain from observing if you are taking any medications to cure an infection, if you are on any hormonal medications, or if you are using any spermicides or lubricants. Here are some guidelines for creating an accurate chart:

1. Wipe your vulva from urethra to anus, and note the sensation of the wipe: dry, smooth or lubricated.
2. Observe the toilet paper for the presence or absence of mucus. Then create your own number coding system to describe the consistency of the mucus. For example: 0 = dry; 1 = damp, but not lubricated; 2 = wet, but not lubricated; 3 = shiny, but not lubricated; 4 = damp and lubricated; 5 = wet and lubricated; 6 = shiny and lubricated.

3. If mucus is present on the toilet paper, finger test it for stretchiness between your thumb and index finger. Again, use a code to describe the consistency: 7 = sticky; 8 = tacky; 9 = stretchy; 10 = pasty; 11 = gummy or gluelike. Using this coding, you can combine numbers to get an accurate picture.

4. Record the numbers you came up with in steps two and three. For example, mucus that is a 5 and 9 is your peak mucus, while a 5 and 10 would represent your cycle past your peak mucus days.

5. Use a coding system to observe the color of the mucus. For example, B = brown; W = white or cloudy; C = clear T = transparent; Y = yellowish or off-white; R = red or pink (your menstrual flow).

6. On your peak days, note how many times you observed your clear, stretchy mucus that day: once, twice, and so on. When you see it a few times a day, it's a good sign.

7. Note the mucus "metamorphosis" pattern. Does it change from clear to cloudy? Clear to dry? Dry to cloudy and then clear?

8. Observe any special circumstances, such as a "double peak," which can happen if you're under stress or have been ill.

9. Take special note of any lower abdominal cramping or backaches. This could be a sign that you're ovulating.

10. Record the length of "stretch" your peak mucus makes. The longer, the better.

But I don't notice any mucus!

This is a problem. Without cervical mucus, sperm can't survive or be transported to the fallopian tubes to fertilize the egg. The mucus also nourishes and protects the sperm, allowing them to live for 3–5 days. If you don't notice any mucus, this is a sign that you may not be ovulating, may have a hormone deficiency, or may even have a vaginal infection of some sort. You'll need to see your doctor to find out why you're not producing mucus. (See chapters 5 and 6 for more details.) That being said, it should also be noted that nothing is 100%. You could still conceive, but a lack of mucus will make conception far more difficult.

The LH Test Kit (The Home Ovulation Test)

Purchase a test kit that will detect your LH surge. This surge triggers ovulation and occurs anywhere from 12 to 36 hours prior to ovulation. This means that you can now accurately pinpoint when you're ovulating 12–36 hours in advance. LH is present in the blood throughout your cycle, but only in small amounts. Just before ovulation, the amount of LH suddenly increases. This test can pick up increased levels of LH in your urine up until 24 hours after your surge. With the aid of a specific kind of antibody, known as *monoclonal antibodies*, these kits can detect even minute amounts of LH in the urine, causing it to turn a specific shade of blue.

Unfortunately, if you have a cycle shorter than 26 days or longer than 33 days, the results of your test may not be as accurate or useful. If you're beginning menopause or are already pregnant (but don't realize it), the results will also be inaccurate.

Since the late 1980s, several LH test kits have come on the market. They take anywhere from 1 to 30 minutes to perform and a variety of brands are available. You can ask either your doctor or pharmacist to recommend one. All LH test kits work on the same principle. You buy the test about 14 days before your next period. Each kit contains a chart that will suggest a good time for you to begin testing, based on the average length of your past periods. Each kit contains either a stick or test pad with a blue reference spot to compare to your test result. Either one will have monoclonal antibodies on them, which will detect any LH. If you're using the stick, you dip the stick into your urine cup and check to see if it changes color; if you're using a test pad, you drop a small amount of your urine onto the pad to see if turns blue. You then continue testing until the blue becomes its darkest shade, which will mark the surge. All kits have an 800 number you can call if you have any questions. However, before you purchase a kit, go over the instructions carefully with either your doctor or pharmacist, and ask if he or she can show you how to use it. The kits are expensive, and the cost depends on how the number of test sticks or test pads (expect either a six-day or nine-day supply). You can also purchase individual refills that cost roughly $10 per refill.

Using the kit along with your mucus observations, menstrual cycle chart, and the BBT chart (discussed below), you should get a very clear picture of your fertility. This kit may also be useful in timing various diagnostic tests (see chapter 5). The following are guidelines for accurate testing:

1. Whether you're leaving a strip stick in a solution or underwater, the timing must be *exact*. Use a stop watch or timer if you have one. (I often stick a cold glass of water in the microwave, turn on the microwave for a specific time, and use *that* for a timer.)
2. Don't drink too many fluids before you collect your urine. It may water down perfectly "surged" urine and give you a false negative reading.
3. Don't reuse your test equipment by trying to wash it out. It won't work.
4. Make sure you check the expiration date on the box before you purchase your kit.
5. Refrain from testing if you have an infection or if you are on medication to treat an in-

fection. Similarly, if you're taking any kind of hormonal concoction, fertility drug (see chapter 7), or steroids (do you have asthma?), don't test. The results won't be accurate.

Basal Body Temperature Chart (Symptothermal Method)

This method is a real nuisance, but it's a good way of charting exactly when you're ovulating. A basal body thermometer (BBT) is an ultrasensitive thermometer that tracks your body's *exact* temperature. A digital thermometer is your best bet. These are fairly cheap and can be purchased at any pharmacy. Each thermometer kit comes with a blank graph that may resemble Figure 3 or Figure 4. These graphs may have space for you to record PMS symptoms. A sample chart, such as the one shown in Figure 5, may also accompany your BBT kit.

Most BBT kits are the same. At the top of the graph are the days of your cycle from 1 to 40, but you add more days if you need to. Underneath each cycle day you write the month and actual calendar date. Vertically listed are temperatures from 99.4°F to 97.0°F. (In Canada, the readings would be in metric units, at from 37.4°C to 36.1°C.)

Each morning, before you get out of bed, you'll need to take your temperature orally (or vaginally, but orally is more accurate) and chart it on the graph. *Unless you take your temperature at the same time each morning, the graph won't be accurate!* After ovulation, your temperature rises between 32 and 32.9 °F (0.2° and 0.5°C). After doing about three charts, you should notice a very distinct pattern of ovulation, which will help you time *future* intercourses and tell you whether you are indeed ovulating regularly. However, this method will not tell you *when* to have intercourse on the spot, since the temperature doesn't rise until *after* ovulation. Yet many couples make the mistake of planning their intercourse around this chart. This is a bad idea and can create stress over sexual intimacy. The purpose of the chart is to help you plan future intercourses and assist you in observing your own unique fertility pattern.

There is debate among gynecologists about the accuracy of these charts. Some women don't experience any sharp differences in temperature, yet are ovulating anyway; some women have an even, or "flat," pattern throughout their cycle, yet are still ovulating. If you're one of them, the absence of a pattern should tell you that you *may* not be ovulating, but *you must also be observing no change in your cervical mucus, and no LH surge from an LH home test kit to suspect that you're anovulatory.* The next step is to have your doctor perform blood tests to check your hormonal levels, or do an *endometrial biopsy* (discussed in chapter 5), a test that determines whether you're ovulating or have a hormonal imbalance.

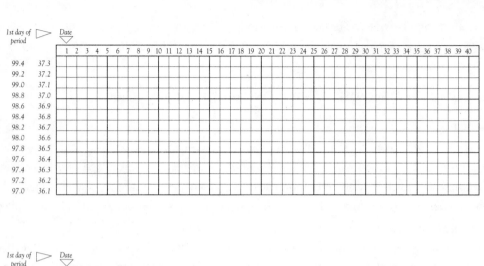

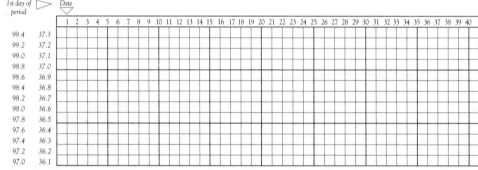

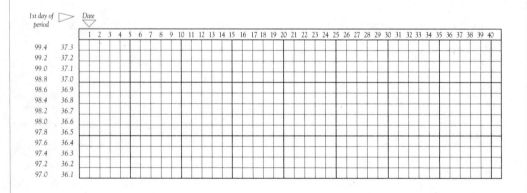

Figure 3.

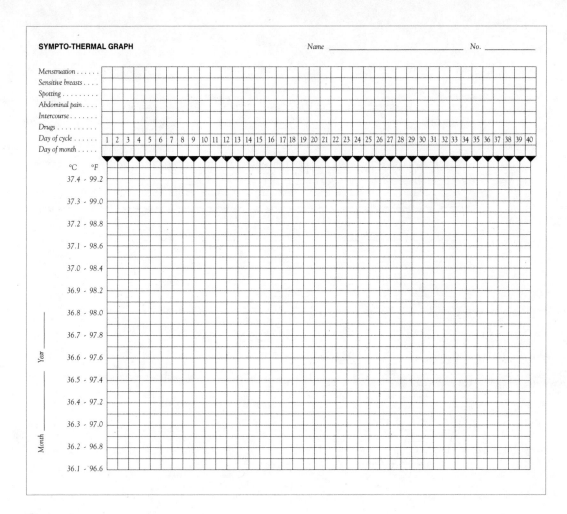

Figure 4.

Reprinted with permission of Serono Canada, Inc., 1994.

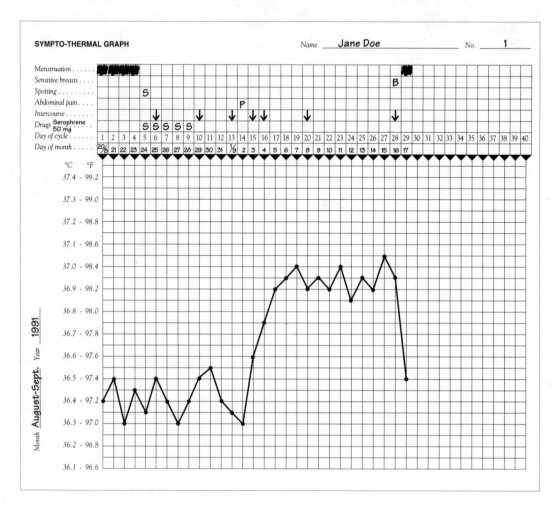

Figure 5.

Reprinted with permission of Serono Canada, Inc., 1994.

Guidelines for an accurate BBT chart

1. The first day of your menstrual flow is day 1 of your BBT chart. Do NOT include spotting prior to your period as day 1. Your temperature should drop when your menstrual flow starts. Record your temperature throughout your period. This information is important.
2. Make sure you note the actual day of the month in the space provided on your chart.
3. Use an oral, digital, basal body thermometer only. A regular thermometer won't do!
4. Take your temperature each morning before you get out of bed. Place the thermometer under your tongue for at least 2–3 minutes.
5. Don't eat, drink, or smoke before you take your temperature (this includes ingesting sperm!)
6. Record your temperature by using a dot, not an X or a checkmark.
7. Use a down-pointing arrow to indicate the days you had intercourse.
8. Record any premenstrual symptoms if there is space on the chart. Otherwise, use your symptom chart to help link a certain temperature to a symptom.
9. Note any special considerations like true illness or fever.
10. Change charts when you get your period again.

Finally, on one of your charts, record what you're eating, how much you're exercising, and whether you're under any unusual stress. Coffee, alcohol, dieting and exercise, and emotional stress all affect your menstrual cycle. By cutting out certain foods or vices, you can see if your menstrual cycle changes.

The BBT Computer

Although the point of doing a BBT chart is to get a visual graph of your cycle, a new product which is a *computerized* BBT thermometer, is now on the market. Known as a BBT computer, this thermometer is essentially designed for the same purposes as an LH surge kit: to predict ovulation for either timing intercourse or various diagnostic tests, discussed in chapter 5.

The way the BBT computer works is similar to any other BBT thermometer, except it flashes a red light during the fertile stage of the cycle and a green light when you're infertile. In order for it to work, you still need to take your temperature daily and at the same time of day. You *can* take the thermometer to the pharmacy and get a printout of your cycle, but critics argue that the point of BBT is for you to do your *own* charting and hence gain control over the rhythms of your cycle. Furthermore, when you do a computer printout, you can't observe symptoms or mucus on the same chart, which critics say is a crucial element in BBT charting.

Attention All Men

Behind every good menstrual chart is an attentive male partner. Help your partner make her observations. Read this chapter, ask her questions, and so on. Help facilitate time for her to do the charting accurately. Sit down with the charts yourself and "proofread" them, making sure that recordings seem accurate.

You can also take part in many observations and even establish a counterchart, observing your partner's premenstrual symptoms such as irritability and weepiness. Ask her to show you her cervical mucus. Test it every day with your own fingers to get to know her pattern. Ask your partner to show you her panties or panty liners so you can observe colors and consistency of mucus. You might ask to look at menstrual discharge to observe the colors and consistencies of the flow. (I know men who do this out of sheer curiosity.) You can also take her temperature and record many of her BBT readings yourself. Finally, you can create a personal chart to observe your own fertility markers.

The Male Fertility Awareness Chart

Pattern a chart after your partner's daily symptom chart and record the following:
1. Ejaculation: Record when you've had an ejaculation on a daily basis, and record the number of ejaculations in any given day. Also note any long periods of abstinence. (Abstinence may place more stress on your prostate gland and affect your ejaculate.)
2. Fevers, colds, and infections: Your sperm count can be affected by illness. Even if you're fighting off a minor infection, increased levels of white blood cells can kill off healthy sperm.
3. If you're not monogamous, record sex you've had with other female (and particularly male) partners. You may need to be tested for STDs.
4. Record any aches or pains in your groin area and any drips or discharge from your urethra.
5. Record any change in your urine color (dark or bloody) and record any burning sensa-

tions in your urethra. This could be a sign of kidney problems, a urinary tract infection, or an inflammation caused by an STD.

6. Record any warts or sores on your genitals. This could be a sign of STDs.

7. Feel your lymph nodes under your ears and around your groin. If they're enlarged, you could be fighting off an infection, which will affect your sperm.

8. Record exposure to high temperatures, such as hot baths, saunas, and sitting in a hot car. This will affect your sperm count (see chapter 2).

9. You, too, should also be recording what you're eating, drinking, and smoking. All these factors can affect your sperm count.

When to Seek Out a Specialist

All this charting should go on for about six months before you start to "try" to conceive. Although it's fine to have as much sex as you like in the beginning, you really won't be able to technically plan your sex by your chart until you have about six cycles' worth of charts.

After your first six charts, your official "trying" phase can begin. You should be having intercourse every other day *around* the time of ovulation. That means you should try a few days before, and keep going until a few days after you ovulate. Women under 35 should try this for about a year. After a year, if you've been unable to get pregnant this way, you should consult your "weed doctor" (see chapter 1) and send your partner off for a semen analysis, detailed in chapter 4. Women over 35 should not wait longer than six months before initiating a fertility investigation. Again, the male partner will need to start the workup process with a semen analysis.

The male workup is the next step when you're not getting pregnant using fertility awareness techniques. This workup usually starts with an initial consultation with your "weed doctor." A fertility specialist is not yet necessary at this point. Bring all six of your charts to your "weed doctor." Make sure your doctor understands your coding methods, and have him or her assess whether you've done the charts accurately. If you haven't, you may need to redo them before an official workup is ordered, but a semen analysis can be done in the meantime just to save time.

In some cases, the charts may reveal an obvious hormonal imbalance that warrants a monitored cycle, or some of the tests discussed in chapter 5. Even if there is an obvious, undisputed female hormonal imbalance, get the semen analysis done *first*. Why? If there is a male factor problem that coexists with the female problem, it will need to be corrected or confirmed anyway, which will save the woman from undergoing a grueling workup. For example, even though your menstrual charts reveal a luteal phase defect, if the male has no sperm at all, fixing the luteal phase defect will do you no good. If the semen analysis is done *first*, the two of you would immediately progress to either donor insemination (see chapter 8), adoption, or making a decision to live childfree (see chapter 10). Time is everything in a fertility investigation. You don't want to waste it.

4

The Male Workup

Infertility has long been perceived as a "woman's problem," even though causes of infertility are evenly split between male and female factors. Yet no matter which partner has the problem, the woman, who ultimately carries the fetus, is often the one who undergoes treatment.

It's impossible to change the basic facts of life, which is why these workups tend to be kinder to men than to women. Delivering numerous sperm samples and possibly urine and blood samples is just about as invasive as it gets for most men. Occasionally, imaging tests and biopsies involving the testicles are needed, but this is not the case in the majority of male workups.

The average, basic female workup consists of invasive, time-consuming procedures, discussed in chapter 5. Understandably, when fertility is in question, the man should *always* be the first to undergo any testing, even if a female factor is suspected. This is because 20% of all infertility involves *both* partners. In this case, if a male factor is untreatable, you can go on as a couple to assisted reproductive technology (ART), which may include donor insemination (see chapter 8) or you can decide on either adoption or childfree living.

This chapter discusses the kinds of tests men will undergo in a fertility investigation and the purpose of each test. To fully explain this, a brief refresher on how the male reproductive organs work and contribute to fertilization is also provided.

Forty-five percent of the time, the male workup will end after one or more normal semen analyses, but it's important for a man to deliver at least two samples, for reasons I'll explain in the next section. An abnormal semen analysis will turn up 55% of the time but 30–40% of the time, no cause for the abnormal semen will be found.

Although the various causes of male factor infertility and the emotional consequences of a diagnosis are covered in this chapter, the treatments are discussed in chapter 6. In many cases, if no treatments may exist for your problem, procedures may be available that can still enable you to *father* a biological child. These procedures may involve *artificial insemination* (AI), *in vitro fertil-*

ization (IVF), or *gamete intrafallopian transfer* (GIFT). If you are not able to father a biological child, there are only three solutions: *donor insemination* (DI), adoption, or childfree living. All ARTs are discussed in chapter 8; alternatives to biological parenting are discussed in chapter 10.

The Semen Factor

Assessing the quality of the semen is the most important aspect of a male workup. Whether the problem is hormonal or structural, all clues to a male factor problem are found within the semen. Before you can grasp exactly what's being analyzed when you deliver that sperm sample, here's a brief refresher on what happens to your sperm from the time they're produced until fertilization. Also, review Figure 6, for a *visual* refresher!

The Sperm Cycle

The a male reproductive hormonal cycle controls semen production. The hormones involved are almost identical to those involved in the female cycle, except that *testosterone* is flooded into the bloodstream instead of estrogen and progesterone. The main difference between the male and female hormonal cycles is that, in the woman, the cycle runs in a continuous loop (see chapter 3), whereas in the man, the cycle runs endlessly without any marked beginning, middle, or end. In women, the ovulation cycle peters out with age, resulting in menopause; in men, there is no time limit for semen production. This distinction in hormonal timing also causes vast differences in male and female sexual behavior, but that's another book!

Every day, a man's testes are busy producing millions of sperm. As in the female cycle, the hypothalamus starts the process by secreting gonadotropin-releasing hormone (GnRH) into the bloodstream. GnRH is released approximately every 90 minutes, triggering the pituitary gland to release both luteinizing hormone (LH) and follicle stimulating hormone (FSH) into the bloodstream, which carries the hormones to the testes. Within the testes, LH goes directly to the *Leydig cells*, which triggers the production of testosterone; FSH goes directly to the *Sertoli cells*, which triggers the production of sperm. When testosterone levels drop, this tells the hypothalamus to release *more* GnRH, which tells the pituitary gland to secrete *more* LH and FSH, which tells the body to make *more* testosterone and sperm. As we discuss later in this chapter, this hormonal interrelationship, clinically called the *hormonal axis*, must be in tip-top shape in order for men to produce enough high-quality sperm to fertil-ize an egg. Trouble with either the Leydig or Sertoli cells may cause unusually high levels of either LH or FSH or unusually low levels of testosterone. Trouble in the hypothalamus or pituitary glands will cause a breakdown of the entire hormonal axis. In all cases, sperm counts will be low or even nonexistent.

The testicles are situated inside the scrotal sac, which is positioned outside the body to keep the tes-ticles at roughly 94°F (35°C), a few degrees cooler than body temperature. The testicles themselves are not visible to the eye and are made up of small, tightly coiled tubes known as *seminiferous tubules*. The sperm are produced inside these tubules, where they stay until they're mature. Sperm cells have their own guardians, the Sertoli cells, also known as nurse cells, which help protect and nourish the sperm until they're mature. These are the cells that respond to FSH. There is one nurse cell for roughly every 150 sperm.

It takes 2–3 months (about 74 days) for sperm

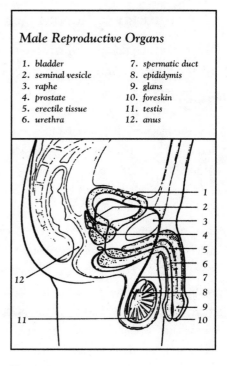

Male Reproductive Organs

1. bladder	7. spermatic duct
2. seminal vesicle	8. epididymis
3. raphe	9. glans
4. prostate	10. foreskin
5. erectile tissue	11. testis
6. urethra	12. anus

Figure 6.
Reprinted with permission of Serono Symposia, USA, 1994

to mature. Mature sperm gather in the center of the tubules, while the immature sperm remain on the outer edges of the tubules. The nurse cells continuously "sweep" sperm into the center as they mature. When the sperm mature, they leave the tubules and enter the *epididymis*, a coiled, tubular organ attached to the testes. Here, the mature sperm learn to "swim" and fine-tune their motility (movement). Mature sperm resemble microscopic tadpoles. They have an enzyme-coated *head*, a *tail*, and a thinner portion of the tail, called an *end piece*.

Once inside the epididymis, mature sperm wait to be ejaculated into the vagina—not unlike the scene depicted in Woody Allen's satirical film, *Everything You Always Wanted to Know About Sex,* where the sperm are waiting to "parachute" out of an aircraft and complete their mission. What happens to the sperm if no ejaculation takes place? They die and are reabsorbed by the body. This is as close as a man comes to having a "period."

Getting Ready to Jump: Ejaculation

The penis is equipped with sensory receptors that tell the brain to make the penis erect. The erectile tissue that lines the penis fills with blood, causing the penis to grow and elongate. The sperm get ejected from the body through one of two parallel sets of tubes, known as the *vas deferens*, an artery that serves as a canal. The vas deferens carries the sperm above the pubic bone, past the bladder. (If you've had a vasectomy, the vas deferens does *not* carry the sperm anywhere, and the sperm are quickly reabsorbed by the body.) The vas deferens takes the sperm to the ejaculatory duct, which serves as a holding area. Until now, the sperm, along with small quantities of fluid (present to help propel the sperm along) are the sole ingredients to the ejaculate. In the holding area, seminal vesicles, small organs nearby, add large quantities of fructose, a sugar solution, to the ejaculate. The fructose nourishes the sperm and turns it into semen. The semen is then dumped into an enlarged section of the urethra called the *bulbous urethra*. The *prostate gland* is connected to the bulbous urethra through a separate duct system. At this point, the prostate gland adds an alkaline fluid to the semen, which will protect it from the acidic environment of the vagina. This, by the way, is the prostate gland's main function in life. A tiny amount of lubricating fluid is then added to the semen by the *Cowper's gland*. The ejaculate is now complete. The fluids are then forcefully ejected by contractions of the pelvic floor muscles and prostate gland. The bladder neck closes to stop sperm from going back into the bladder. An average ejaculate contains 40 million to 150 million sperm, out of which only a few hundred will even come *close* to the egg. The semen measures between a half to a full teaspoon and is ejaculated through the urethra. (To the naked eye, semen without sperm is indistinguishable from semen with sperm, which is why males who produce little or no sperm do not realize it.)

Survival of the Fittest: Fertilization

Once inside the vagina, the semen immediately coagulates, for reasons not yet understood. Because the vagina is acidic, only about 10% of the sperm will survive the first 10 minutes inside the vagina. After about 20 minutes, the semen becomes fluid again, enabling the surviving sperm to swim up the reproductive tract. Here's where the cervical mucus enters the picture. When a portion of the surviving sperm reach the cervical mucus, they will find tiny strands of protein within it that will carry them toward the uterus. *This protein is present only in midcycle mucus, which has an egg-white consistency.* The mucus is a sign that ovulation has just taken place or will be taking place shortly. The woman's egg remains viable for about 12–24 hours; the sperm can live up to 48–72 hours. This creates a reproductive window of roughly four days.

As discussed in chapter 2, new research indicates that when a woman reaches orgasm at the *time* of ejaculation (but not before), her orgasmic contractions also help to propel the sperm upward, toward the uterus. However, if a woman reaches orgasm prior to ejaculation (during foreplay, for example), the contractions may help to keep the sperm away.

Once the sperm reach the uterus and continue upward, they number in the hundreds. Some of this sperm will get lost or will become embedded in the lining of the fallopian tubes. The enzyme cap that coats the head of the sperm is covered with a net of membranes that protect it. This membrane is almost completely worn away by this point, so when the sperm reaches the egg, the enzymes are "naked" and can easily penetrate the egg. During many of the assisted conception procedures discussed in chapter 8, this membrane is artificially worn away through a process known as *sperm washing*. The clinical term for this membrane wear and tear is known as the *capacitation process*.

When the sperm enters the egg's outer layer, a biochemical change in the egg takes place, making it impossible for any other sperm to penetrate it. The sperm and the egg at this point merge genetic material. The entire fertilization process takes about 24 hours, and the fertilized egg takes about four days to reach the uterus. The egg then secretes a hormone called *human chorionic gonadotropin* (HCG). In a home pregnancy test kit, this hormone causes the stick to change color.

Sometimes the egg will not travel to the uterus to develop, but will instead grow inside the fallopian tube. This is known as an *ectopic, or tubal pregnancy*, and is more common in women who have a history of sexually transmitted diseases (STDs) or intrauterine device (IUD) use.

Rarely, some freakish versions of fertilization can result in a *molar pregnancy*, where there is either no developing embryo or an embryo that will not be able to survive at birth. There are three ways this can occur: two sperm can fertilize one egg, with the loss of the mother's chromosomes; one sperm can enter the egg and then divide, delivering a double dose of chromosomes to the egg instead of its usual single dose; or an abnormal sperm carrying two sets of chromosomes can fertilize the egg.

The Semen Analysis

As discussed in chapter 1, when you and your partner suspect infertility, the semen analysis begins the workup for both of you. A normal *series* of semen analyses will prompt a female workup; an abnormal series will prompt a male workup. This test can be handled by your primary care doctor, your partner's gynecologist, or your own urologist or andrologist. In short, whoever has been handling your preconception screenings and "weedings" until this point will manage the semen analyses.

This same doctor should also ask you questions about your medical/surgical history and perform a thorough physical exam, including an examination of your external genitals. This helps the doctor rule out infection, structural abnormalities, and so on. The doctor may order general lab tests to rule out other diseases, such as a urine test for diabetes or kidney infection; blood tests for complete blood counts, ruling out syphilis, anemia, or leukemia; and screenings to rule out viral or bacterial infections. Your doctor should also do a thyroid function test. In general, bloodwork is not routine, however.

You should also be asked about your sex life: how old you were when you reached puberty, first erections, viral infections after puberty (such as mumps or high fevers), previous paternity, how often you have intercourse, how often you masturbate, whether you use lubricants, whether you have any of the lifestyle habits discussed in chapter 2 that may interfere with your fertility. Sometimes this more probing look at your personal life isn't done unless your semen analysis is *abnormal,* or unless you're referred to a urologist or andrologist. Detailed physical exams of the testes, and rectal exams that evaluate the prostate gland and seminal vesicles, aren't done unless you're referred to a urologist.

If you have diabetes or (had) testicular cancer

After you produce your semen sample, ask your doctor to perform a *urinalysis* (urine test) *next.* A common problem for men with these conditions is *retrograde ejaculation,* where the ejaculate is propelled backward into the bladder. Men with diabetes may gradually lose nerve function at the bladder's opening, causing sperm to shoot backward during ejaculation. Men who have had lymph nodes removed in the testicles may have nerve damage that may interfere with the closing of the bladder neck during ejaculation.

In these cases, semen would be present in your urine. In order to diagnose retrograde ejaculation, you must collect your urine immediately *after* an ejaculation. Doing the urinalysis first can save you a lot of time. Occasionally, antihistamines may improve sperm ejaculation because they help to close the sphincter muscle between the urethra and the bladder.

Otherwise, while there is no specific treatment for retrograde ejaculation, there is a procedure your doctor can do that will enable you to biologically father a child. It involves extracting live sperm from your urine and then depositing it into your partner. Success rates for this procedure are high. (See chapter 6 for more details.)

You *can* do this test at home. Once your doctor gives you a requisition for a semen analysis, you can take the requisition to any lab. All labs are equipped with take-home semen analysis kits. As long as you live within a half-hour drive of the lab, you can produce the sample at home and drop it off at the lab. Sperm can survive for at least that long in the cup. It's important to keep the specimen warm. Placing it in a front pants pocket, tucking it into the waistline of your pants, or tucking it under your arm is the best way to transport it. If you spill any of the semen during or after collection, you'll need to repeat the test. Do *not* put the collection in the fridge or freezer overnight.

The kit includes some of the instructions I'll go into below, perhaps a small questionnaire with your name, address, insurance information, and some brief medical history questions, and a *sterile* specimen cup. (A clean glass jar is also fine, but don't go the Dixie cup route.) If your doctor has a laboratory in his or her office building or clinic, you could produce your sperm sample in the office bathroom or another private room. This is certainly the simplest route.

Guidelines for good samples

You'll need to wait at least two full days after your last ejaculation to do the test.

If you've taken any medications (such as antibiotics, for example) prior to the test, you'll need to wait at least four months after you swallow your last pill before you can produce a sample. It can take three to four months for your sperm count to come back to normal levels. You can either masturbate into the specimen cup, or your partner can bring you to orgasm through petting. Some labs tell you it's fine for your partner to help you ejaculate via oral sex or coitus interruptus (pulling out), but saliva or vaginal mucus may interfere with the test results. If you're doing it through intercourse, don't use collected sperm from a regular condom. There are special condoms that may be used, known as "semen collection devices" (SCDs). Your doctor can tell you where to purchase them. If you are masturbating, avoid using creams or lubricants because they can poison the sperm.

What's normal?

There are several elements your doctor will look for in your lab results. *Because semen is extremely volatile and changes daily, you'll need to deliver at least three semen specimens so your lab can establish a semen baseline.* Since numbers and percentages vary from man to man, sample to sample, minimal limits of "normal" have been set. Your sample needs to meet these limits on at least two occasions to be truly considered a "normal" result. *Warning: If your doctor sends you off for a female workup after only one normal semen analysis, you should seek a second opinion or request that your doctor order another semen analysis.* If your doctor is satisfied that you're "normal" after only one sample, this indicates that your doctor doesn't know what he of she is doing. Two normal semen analyses are enough proof that you're indeed "normal."

On the flip side, if your sample comes back "abnormal" the first try, don't accept this finding until you do at least another test. Two abnormal semen analyses that are *consistent* are enough proof that there's a problem. If no sperm was found in your sample, immediately request that your doctor do a urinalysis to rule out retrograde ejaculation.

The semen analysis checks for a few things:

- *Sperm count.* There is debate among the medical community about what a healthy number of sperm is. The World Health Organization (WHO) considers 20 million sperm per milliliter to be fertile; the International Society of Andrology (ISA) consider 40 million sperm per milliliter to be fertile. Generally, anything below 20 million is considered a low sperm count. Anything between 20 and 100 million sperm is considered normal. Keep in mind, however, that sperm numbers can change daily, weekly, and monthly. Colds, flus, STDs, infections, antibiotics, temperature, and ejaculation frequencies all will affect the number. Also keep in mind that men with sperm counts of well below 20 million have often been able to father children.

- *Motility.* This refers to the sperm's ability to swim and move quickly. Again, infection, illnesses, or gonadotoxins such as marijauna or tobacco can affect movement. Just because the sperm are produced in high numbers and are shaped well doesn't mean they're all on the Olympic swim team. Motility is one of the most important determining factors in the sperm's ability to fertilize the egg. At least 60% of your sperm need to be motile in order to be considered "normal." At least 65% of the sperm must be alive. They also need to be moving *forward.* When you find out your motility percentage, this is the percentage of sperm that are moving. For example, 75% motility means that 75% of your sperm are moving.

- *Morphology.* This refers to the shape and maturity of the sperm cells to determine the quality, *viscosity of semen* (consistency—thickening is a bad sign), *volume of semen* (amount of semen produced—about 1 teaspoonful is normal), and the *pH balance* (it should be slightly alkaline). Some examples of poor morphology would be large numbers of sperm with two heads, no tails, two tails, no heads, deformed tails and heads, and so on. Again, infection and gonodatoxins can affect morphology, and again, at least 60% of your sperm need to be formed normally in order to meet the "limits of adequacy." Your volume needs to reach between 1.5 and 5 cubic centimeters in order to meet these same limits.

- *Clumping.* Sperm that clump together are unhealthy and could be a sign of *immunological infertility*, in which your body is making antisperm antibodies.
- *White blood cell count.* High levels of white blood cells in the semen may indicate infection. Treatment for infections ranging from *prostatitis* (inflammation of the prostate gland) to *orchitis* (inflammation of the testes) is discussed in chapter 6.
- *Red blood cell count.* High levels of red blood cells in the semen aren't normal. You'll need to be evaluated for underlying conditions such as infections.

Finding out the results

A significant percentage of all semen analyses will have flaws in them. Men tend to be more in the dark about their test results than women, who usually have some symptoms that hint at a problem. Men usually have no symptoms that would indicate male infertility, whereas women often experience pain or irregular cycles that indicate a female factor.

If you don't hear from your doctor's office within two weeks after your test, you can assume that the results are normal. The results are categorized into two basic groupings: normal or abnormal. You should also request a copy of the lab report so you can study it yourself and ask questions about terminology you don't understand. Having a copy of the report will allow you to make copies for the next specialist(s) you encounter. (Don't count on your doctor to send the results.) A normal test series ends the male workup here. You and your partner will then go on as a couple to a gynecologist and/or reproductive endocrinlogist to begin the female workup.

An abnormal test could involve any one of the above categories. You could also have sperm that meet the limits in one category but not the other. For example, you could have excellent motility but a low sperm count. In this case, you would not be classified as subfertile, which means you're not as fertile as you could be. Many men make the assumption that a diagnosis of being subfertile is the same as being infertile. *This is not true.* A subfertile faces *lower odds* of conceiving a child in any *one* cycle. This is quite different than being infertile, which is a complete inability to father a child. For example, if a normal couple has a 20% chance of conceiving each month, subfertile men have *less* than a 20% chance of conceiving each month. As one urologist told me, "It's like Las Vegas. If you roll the dice often enough, most of the subfertile couples will conceive. It may just take longer."

If your results came back showing you produced no sperm at all, a condition known as *azoospermia*, all categories in the sperm analysis would be affected, and you would be considered infertile. A diagnosis of azoospermia must always be followed up by a urinalysis to rule out retrograde ejaculation. Again, don't accept this diagnosis until two more semen analyses confirm it. In other cases, abnormalities may be found in several categories, such as motility, morphology, and volume, while the sperm count may be normal.

If after three collections your results are indeed abnormal, you'll be referred to a urologist and/or andrologist for further diagnostic tests. Before initiating more complicated lab work, though, your specialist will have you repeat the semen analysis at least twice over a three-month period. Again, fevers, infections, or viruses can affect the sperm count for months afterward. If two more collections come back abnormal, the male workup continues and will now focus on discovering why your results are abnormal.

Statistically, most male infertility revolves around structural problems. Roughly 40% of all male infertility is due to *varicoceles*, a varicose vein in the leg that moves up into the scrotum. Two to three percent of all male infertility is due to obstructions (blockage). Out of this group, 5% of the obstructions are in the ejaculatory ducts, 2–3% is due to post-testis obstruction ("bad plumbing"), and 95% of the time, the blockage occurs in the epididymis. In these cases, microsurgery can remedy the problem (see chapter 6). About 10% of all male inferlity is caused by infections. About 5% of all male infertility is caused by immunological problems, where your body produces antisperm antibodies that kill off the sperm. About 2% of male infertility is due to hormonal factors, while another 5% of all male infertility is caused by various anatomical defects, such as torsion or undescended testicles, discussed in chapter 6. The remaining percentage is caused by a hodgepodge of genetic problems (discussed below), congenital abnormalities (covered in chapter 6), and retrograde ejaculation.

Finding the Cause

Investigating male factor infertility works differently than most diagnostic processes because, you have a diagnosis *before* you have the cause. With other diseases, the diagnosis is made when the cause behind your symptoms is *found*. When you're referred to either a urologist and/or andrologist, your abnormal semen analysis report will have at least one of these diagnostic labels:

- Low sperm count: *oligospermia*
- Poor motility: *asthenospermia*
- Poor morphology: *teratospermia*
- No sperm: *azoospermia*
- High white blood cell count: *pyospermia*

The next test you undergo will depend greatly on your lab report. Since most explained male infertility (vs. unexplained) is structural in origin, common structural problems such as varicoceles or blockages may sought out first.

Finding Varicoceles

If all your sperm characteristics are abnormal, chances are the culprit is a *varicocele* (varicose vein in the testicle). Any experienced urologist or andrologist (and some primary care physicians) can find this common structural problem, which afflicts 15% of the male population and accounts for at least 40% of all male factor infertility. Usually the doctor can find a varicocele just by feeling your scrotum with his or her fingers. In fact, 80% of all varicoceles are discovered this way. You'll need to be in a standing position for several minutes before your doctor can find them, however. If a varicocele is suspected, you may need to have either an ultrasound done via a Doppler ultrasonic stethoscope, or a *venography*, which is an X ray of your testicular veins, to confirm the diagnosis. In a venography, a contrast dye is injected into the renal vein outlining the spermatic vein to see how well the blood flows around the testes. *Scrotal thermography*, which uses infrared to detect temperature gradients in the testicles, can also confirm a varicocele. In some cases, varicoceles are too small to palpitate by hand.

Varicocele is a particularly common problem for men who are experiencing secondary infertility, where they have already fathered one or more children but cannot father additional children. Varicoceles cause low sperm counts and poor morphology and may even interfere with testosterone levels. Varicoceles are treatable with microsurgery and are discussed further in chapter 6. Pregnancy rates typically soar from 6% per year prior to treatment to 40% per year after treatment.

Finding Other Anatomical Problems

As your doctor feels your penis, scrotum, and testicles for firmness and size, he or she will be able to detect less common anatomical problems immediately, such as *torsion*, where one testicle is twisted, inflammation, where one or both testicles may be infected (*orchitis*); undescended testicles, and other congenital problems (see chapter 6). During this exam, honest answers to tough questions may also help to pinpoint sexual disorders that interfere with ejaculation.

Checking Out Azoospermia and Oligospermia

Azoospermia or oligospermia are often caused by structural problems that exist within the seminal vesicles and testes. In azoospermia, the first step is always a urinalysis to rule out retrograde ejaculation. Normal seminal vesicles should also add fructose to the semen. When there's no sign of fructose, this indicates that there's a problem with the vas deferens or seminal vesicles, or it could also be a sign of retrograde ejaculation. Fructose in semen with *no* sperm indicates a variety of other structural problems that could be at work: blockage in the ejaculatory ducts, a cyst in the pouch of the prostate, or an inflamed prostate gland. Problems within the seminal vesicles or the prostate gland are confirmed by a thorough *digital rectal exam*, possibly followed by a *vasography*. This is an X ray of sperm transport ducts. Radio-opaque dye is injected into the vas deferens and ejaculatory ducts, and then an X ray of the dye flowing through the tubes is taken. This test is similar to the *hysterosalpingogram* performed on women (see chapter 5). The vasography results confirm blockage, which may be repaired through surgical techniques.

Hormonal testing

If no structural problem is found, there could be a hormonal imbalance at work. Simple blood tests will check your FSH, LH, prolactin, and testosterone levels, giving your doctor a clear picture of the hormonal axis. For example, high levels of FSH mean that there's trouble within the seminiferous tubules, where the Sertoli cells live. One of the most common male endocrine problems is to find normal levels of LH and testosterone but very high levels of FSH. High levels of FSH is the body's way of shouting at the seminifeous tubules, telling them to WORK!

When your FSH levels are too high and your testosterone levels are low, this is testicular failure; there is no treatment. Donor insemination, adoption, or childfree living are your only options.

High levels of LH indicate problems with the Leydig cells, which make all the androgens, including testosterone. Although Leydig cell problems are almost always associated with a sperm-producing problem, sperm-producing problems rarely involve the Leydig cell. Levels of androgens and estrogens need to be checked as well.

When levels of either FSH or LH (and consequently testosterone) are low, it's a sign that there is a pituitary gland problem. This can be remedied with fertility drugs. Human menopausal gonadotropin (HMG) (Pergonal), which is pure FSH, can be used to stimulate the seminiferous tubules, or clomiphene citrate (CC) (Clomid), which is pure LH, can stimulate the Leydig cells. Both these drugs are discussed in chapter 7.

Sometimes *hyperprolactinemia* is the culprit. This is more commonly a problem in women, but men may have high prolactin levels due to a benign tumor in the pituitary gland, which will interfere with testosterone levels. This tumor can be removed, or the drug *bromocriptine* (discussed in chapter 7), may be prescribed to block prolactin secretions.

In more extreme cases, *hypogonodatrophic hypogonadism* may be discovered. Here, very low levels of FSH and LH with possibly normal testosterone levels may be found. This means that there is no hormone stimulation taking place at all, causing no testicular or sperm development. This problem is usually caught well before a man ever considers children, because he will remain boylike. He will have small testes, have missed puberty, and have extremely low levels of FSH and LH. This disorder indicates *Kallmann's syndrome* (curiously, these men also lack the ability to smell). Hormone injections will take care of the problem. If, for some reason, this syndrome was never diagnosed, it is usually detected during a physical exam.

Thyroid disorders are also common hormonal culprits. Your thyroid gland is responsible for maintaining cell function throughout your body. When your thyroid is overstimulated (hyperthyroidism) or understimulated (hypothyroidism), the result can be a low sperm count and poor libido. This problem is easily treated by an endocrinologist.

Genetic testing

Genetic testing is often done if no sperm are found. Here, a chromosome (karyotype) study is done on a blood sample. This study will reveal possible defects, such as Klinefelter's syndrome, where a man carries an extra X chromosome, resulting in no sperm within semen and no sperm production in the testes. Some men have mosaic Klinefelter's syndrome, in which some cells are normal, and others have an extra X chromosome. Although these men may have some sperm, they are usually infertile. Klinefelter's syndrome afflicts one in four hundred men—not as uncommon as you may think.

Young's syndrome is another genetic disorder of the *cilia*, small hairs that exist throughout bodily tubes and ducts. Men with Young's syndrome will have no sperm as well as respiratory problems. Here, the epididymis gets plugged up with mucus, which normally is cleaned by the cilia. The lungs will be blocked because of a mucus plug as well. *Intracytoplasmic sperm injection* (ICSI), a "hybrid" of *in vitro fertilization* (IVF), can be used in these cases to help produce offspring. (See chapter 8 for details.)

The testicular biopsy

This is the procedure men fear the most when they hear the phrase *infertility testing*. When there's no sperm, but all the diagnostic tests seem to check out normally, a testicular biopsy is an important part of the male workup. This biopsy will determine whether the problem originates in the sperm *production* process or sperm *transport* system.

To have the biopsy done, you'll report to the hospital as a day patient and undergo either a

Testicular biopsy

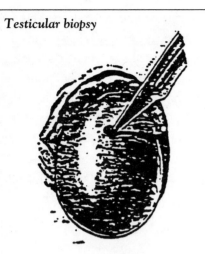

A. *After a small incision is made in the scrotal skin, an incision is made into the testicle through which the tubules protrude.*

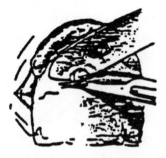

B. *Extruded tubules are removed. They are placed in a special solution and examined microscopically. The small incisions in the testicle and scrotum are then closed with absorbable sutures.*

Figure 7.
Reprinted with permission of Serono Symposia, USA, 1994

general or local anesthetic. During the procedure, a small piece of testicular tissue, which contains both the seminifirous tubules (which house the Sertoli cells) and the Leydig cells, is removed so it can be examined by a pathologist (see figure 7). You're then sewn up with stitches that gradually dissolve into the body. The procedure takes 15–30 minutes, and you'll be able to go home the same day. This is considered *very* minor surgery, and the only post-operative side effect you'll likely experience is some pain and tenderness, which a painkiller will take care of. Very rarely, some men may experience bleeding or swelling, usually caused by an infection in the incision.

There are four common results to a testicular biopsy. "Normal" means that your testicles are operating just fine and are producing healthy sperm, but there is an obstructed or missing duct leading from the testicle to the prostate. This abnormality is preventing the sperm from getting into the ejaculate. Microsurgery techniques can be used to treat an epididymal obstruction, and sperm aspiration can be done when there are absent ducts. Endoscopic surgery can be performed if there is an obstruction in the ejaculatory ducts.

"Maturation arrest patterns" means that your seminiferous tubules, which contain the Sertoli cells that nurse the sperm, aren't working properly. Something stops the sperm from developing into fully normal, mature sperm. This may be treated with medications. When hypospermatogenesis is found, it means that there are also problems within the seminiferous tubules. Here, while sperm are produced, the number of normal sperm produced represent a small fraction. Sometimes a hormonal imbalance is behind this, which may be treatable. Often the causes are *idiopathic*, meaning "we don't know."

"Germinal cell aplasia" means that your testicles do not have the germ cells within them that produce the sperm. (Both the sperm and egg start out in the body as tiny germ cells, which then go through a maturing and dividing process.) There is no known cause of this, and there is no treatment available. Options in this case are donor insemination (see chapter 8), adoption, or childfree living (see chapter 10).

Other results biopsy may find problems within the Leydig cell, indicating a testosterone deficiency, evidence of inflammation or infection of the testicles, or, *very* rarely, cancer, which interferes with sperm production. It's important to remember that a testicular biopsy is never performed as a first procedure and is reserved for situations where every other possible diagnostic test for an absent sperm count has been exhausted.

Checking Out Asthenospermia, Teratospermia, and Pyospermia

When sperm counts are normal but motility and morphology are poor, your work-up will move in a slightly different direction. The first step is to rule out varicoceles, discussed above. If no varicoceles are found, infection is the next best explanation, particularly when poor motility is the *only* factor. In short, when something goes wrong *inside* the sperm, something *outside* is usually the culprit. Infections that affect motility are varied, ranging from the gamut of STDs to garden-variety flus and colds. To detect infections, cultures of the semen, urine, and possibly fluid from the prostate gland will be sent to a laboratory for examination. In some studies, up to 10% of infertile men have infections but show no symptoms of infection. In women, untreated bacterial infections almost always head for the fallopian tubes, causing the majority of structural problems that affect female fertility; in men, untreated bacterial infections tend to head for the prostate gland, causing prostatitis. Bladder infections (cystitis) in both men and women will also affect fertility. Treating infections is covered in chapter 6.

Whether you're infection-free or not, you'll proceed to a sperm antibody test (via blood test and semen sample) to explore whether *immunological infertility* is a possible cause of your poor motility/morphology or even a consequence of an infection. Sometimes an injury or infection can cause your immune system to react to itself, creating an autoimmune response, which means "self-attacking." Here, the immune system somehow recognizes the sperm as an invader and forms antibodies to it that coat the sperm and ultimately kill them off. This is often a cause of poor motility or visible clumping. Men who have had vasectomy reversals are particularly vulnerable to this, and men who have ingested their own sperm are now recognized as "high risk" for immunological infertility (see chapter 2).

Genetic testing may be the next step if you're infection free. Another genetic defect, *immotile cilia syndrome*, is diagnosed when the sperm tail cannot propel the sperm forward. Here, the sperm count may be high, but the motility would be very poor. Treatment is not available for this defect.

Unexplained Infertility

Many men who produce abnormal semen analyses will find out the cause of their *whateverspermia*. In 30–40% of the cases, no definite cause behind semen abnormalities will be discovered, but doctors usually will be able to speculate or at least tell you what part of the body is not working.

About 10–20% of all men with a normal semen analysis series will go on with their partners to a female workup, which will include a *postcoital test* (PCT—you have intercourse, she goes to the doctor) that checks whether your sperm is able to penetrate your partner's cervical mucus. The PCT also makes sure that your partner isn't making antisperm antibodies, killing your sperm once they're in the vagina. After all the female tests, these men may discover that nothing is wrong with their partners either. This is called *unexplained infertility* (or *idiopathic infertility*). In this case, there may be a problem with the sperm's ability to penetrate the egg—something that would *not* show up in a semen anaylsis or in any of the female tests.

Just to be thorough, your doctor may suggest a *sperm penetration assay* (SPA) or *hamster-egg penetration test* (via semen sample). It's important to have this test done if you have a low sperm count and are planning IUI or IVF, or if you're planning to do IVF for other reasons.

The test takes a million washed, mature sperm (i.e., "capacitated") and leaves them to incubate with 20–25 hamster eggs. These eggs have had their outer shells removed to allow penetration but *no* development. (Don't worry—your genetic material will *not* turn up in an unsuspecting hamster!) Your doctors can determine the fertile potential of the sperm by observing how many eggs were penetrated. This test is not usually routine in a normal male workup. The test was originally developed in 1979 and since then has undergone many upgrades. A positive result (meaning yes, your sperm can penetrate) is usually reliable, but some false negatives have been reported, where the test reveals that the sperm is unable to penetrate the egg, yet a pregnancy has resulted nonetheless.

The Male Factor Roller Coaster

During the workup, most men may feel isolated in the doctor's waiting room, which is filled mostly with women. Men who choose to deliver their samples at the office may dread the room, where they must produce their sample. These rooms usually have a variety of *Penthouse* magazines and assorted porn videos to speed the process along. Why are there so *many* women in the waiting room if infertility is split between male and female factors? Many of those women are there for treatment after a male factor problem has been discovered; many of those women are there to get sperm requisitions and test kits to take home to their partners, who are doing all of their workup tests at home; and some may be *single* and pursuing a family through donor insemination.

Every infertility situation is unique and therefore carries unique emotional and social consequences. When it is a female factor problem, men tend to play the "supportive partner" role, allowing their partners time to grieve, time to rant and rave, time to cry, and time to be angry. They will also reassure their female partners about their attractiveness and femininity. But few men will truly *feel* a female factor problem, although they obviously will be affected by it.

When a couple is dealing with a male factor problem, women who star in the "supporting role" tend to hit a brick wall. Many men will go the "ostrich" route, preferring *not* to discuss the problem, *not* to reveal their true feelings, and hence *not* to plan for an alternative, such as donor insemination or adoption. Many will experience depression and even sexual dysfunction as a result. Many men will turn to addictions such as work or alcohol.

The urge to repress feelings is a male tendency that is encouraged not only by our social structures and definitions of "masculinity," but often by male friends and acquaintances. After interviewing many couples who have dealt with male factor infertility, the number-one problem most men faced was admitting their fertility to another *male*, particularly close family members and friends. Psychologists and psychiatrists substantiate the finding. The psychiatric literature confirms that while women focus on the loss of a baby, putting to rest their dreams of pregnancy, childbirth, and breastfeeding, men focus on their fears of *competition*: "What will my friends say?" As a result, many men will choose silence over disclosure.

This is an understandable but emotionally unhealthy choice. In the long run, continued silence will create communication gaps in your relationship with your partner. Admitting the infertility to even one other male will help you find a "place" for your feelings. To help you break that silence, I've compiled a list of guidelines based on the experiences of many men and couples who have dealt with male factor infertility. Not one male I spoke with regretted his disclosure.

Guidelines for Breaking the Silence

1. *What are you afraid of?* Try to imagine your worst fears of disclosure: being the subject of cruel jokes at the office; being ostracized by the "guys"; being laughed at by people you respect. Try to evaluate whether your fears are justified, and think about how your lifestyle would change if these fears were actualized. For example, if your best friend laughed at the problem, this information could help you re-evaluate your criteria for friends and help you form more lasting, deeper friendships. Male factor infertility tends to be like a wedding or funeral: It brings out the worst and best in people.

2. *Educate yourself.* Request literature, article clippings or videos from your doctor on male infertility. If this fails, do your own research through organizations and libraries. The more you read about your particular problem, the less isolated and freakish you'll feel.

3. *A date for discussion.* Make a date with your partner to discuss your problem. Clear a night on your calendar and *devote* the evening to discussing your feelings and options. The more your partner feels included in your pain, the more she can support you rather than just "guess" at how you must be feeling. You can also use your partner to practice disclosure lines on other males or family members. For example, ask her advice on how to start: "There's something I need to tell you," "I'm telling you this because I think you'll understand," and so on. Ask her advice on comeback lines to rude comments such as "When are you two having a baby?" or male friends who joke, "You can't use *my* sperm!"

4. *Start a journal.* Write down your feelings instead of keeping them inside. Your journal will begin to feel like an old friend, help you sort out your feelings, and help you *monitor* them from month to month. Are you coping better today than last month? Are your coping skills getting worse? You can even read your journal entries to your partner. Or, if you're not able to talk to her, you may want to invite her to read the journal anytime she wishes. (See figure 8 for an example of journal notes between a real-life couple coping with male infertility.)

5. Find a good *male* friend. You need to talk to another man about your infertility. If you don't have a male friend or close family member (brother, brother-in-law, father, cousin) you can talk to, maybe you need to rethink some of your relationships. Try to choose someone who poses no threat to you regarding workplace or community politics. Take some time to find this person. Don't rush it. All you need is one good friend. (See #6.)

6. *Seek out a male counselor.* Again, the idea is to find another male to confide in. Someone

who knows what it's like to *own* a penis and testes may be able to offer you more practical solutions to your dilemma. You don't have to sign up for long-term counseling; just a few sessions with a male social worker or male psychologist should do. In some cases, male clergy can make ideal counselors.

7. *Find a good support group.* All major cities have branches of infertility support organizations. You need to find other couples in your situation and hear that other men have felt what you do now. This may be where you find that one good friend to talk to.

As discussed at the beginning of this chapter, 45% of all men will graduate to a female workup after three normal semen analyses. The next chapter may be in order or out of order, depending on the results of your male workup. For treatment options to many male factor problems, see chapters 6 and 8. Donor insemination is covered in chapter 8.

Notes between a couple dealing with male infertility

WHY SHOULD I BELIEVE IN HIM?

(expletive)

WHAT GOOD CAN COME OF THIS?

Damn what prevents me from being a father.

I am so (expletive) angry

Figure 8a.

Source: Infertility Awareness Association of Canada, 1994

He has taken a part of me that means the most.
I want a child. I want a baby . . . that will never be part of
me—THERE CAN NEVER BE A PART OF ME THAT
CONTINUES, a fact that can never be denied, I can not
handle the thought that I will not continue . . . my eyes,
my thoughts, my dreams. I will never have the joy or the
satisfaction of saying "this is a part of me." Yet, I see
the cruelty of so many parents towards their children!
Children they have never even thought of as a privilege.
(Expletive) THEM FOR NOT LOVING THEIR OFFSPRING
ENOUGH . . . I'm angry and very mad at God.
He has taken the one thing I would have loved
unconditionally.

Figure 8b.
Source: Infertility Awareness Association of Canada, 1994

Dearest P.,

I'm so sorry you went through what you were feeling last night. It pains me to see you unhappy.

I'm sure you know that I understand and share your anger. I'm sure you also know that you are already an important part of our children. You may not be able to give them the shape of their eyes, the curve of their nose or their beautiful thick hair, but you will give them things much more important—the shape of their beliefs, share curiosity and compassion are just a few of the things that come to mind as I picture you sharing your joy of life with them.

P., you are <u>very</u> special and I look forward to having your children.

Love always,

S.

xo

Figure 8c.

Source: Infertility Awareness Association of Canada, 1994

5

The Female Workup

After your male partner has delivered two normal semen analyses, the two of you can proceed to the female workup. The female workup is infamous for its involved and invasive testing. Many of the tests require a woman to be at a certain phase of her cycle, which can result in weeks between tests and months before a reason for your infertility is found. For 10–20% of infertile couples, no fertility problem will be identified after the female workup, leaving you with the maddening diagnosis of unexplained infertility, discussed below, and in detail in chapter 6. The good news is that there is still a 70–90% chance that the cause of your infertility *will* be found during this workup.

About 30% of all female infertility is caused by hormonal factors. This is a significant percentage when you consider that only 5% of all male factor infertility is hormonal. As a result, a great deal of female factor infertility can be treated with medications. The remaining 50–60% of all female factor infertility is caused by structural problems involving infections or inflammations of the fallopian tubes or other pelvic organs. When this is the case, there are several microsurgical procedures that can repair these problems. If repair surgery is not possible in your case, you'll need to look at other options: treatment asissted reproductive technology (ART), adoption, or childfree living. This chapter focuses on all the *diagnostic* tests involved with the female workup and discusses the appropriate procedures from least invasive to most invasive. Treatment, when available, for female factor infertility is covered in chapter 6, fertility drugs are addressed in chapter 7, and ART techniques are detailed in chapter 8.

Some women will still require a full workup even though a male factor problem has already been identified. This is because the woman is the one who will need to undergo the bulk of ART treatments. In addition, in 20% of the cases, both partners have problems. A fertility doctor will need to know whether the woman is *able* to conceive via intrauteriane insemination (IUI), in vitro fertilization (IVF), gamete intrafallopian transfer (GIFT), or even donor insemination (DI). As a result, this chapter introduces an option that I'll explore further in chapter 10: *refusing treatment.*

What's the First Step?

Your primary care physician will refer you to a gynecologist who subspecializes in reproductive endocrinology. Review chapter 1, which covers guidelines for finding a good specialist and the questions you need to ask. If your gynecologist has been managing the workup so far and is skilled in reproductive endocrinology, you don't need to be referred elsewhere.

Both partners should see the gynecologist together. You should also bring in your basal body temperature (BBT) charts, and any other charts you're using to keep track of your cycles (see chapter 3). The doctor will begin by interviewing both of you. *Note: To save time, bring along your medical chart from the initial male workup and physical, as well as the results from the last three semen analyses. Otherwise, men may wind up doing everything again!*

The doctor may even request *separate* interviews, asking each of you about your relationship, how long you've been together, and how long you've been trying to conceive. A man will be asked whether he has impregnated a woman in the past; a woman will be asked whether she has ever been pregnant, has had any abortions, or has had previous pelvic surgery. These questions help the doctor determine the likelihood of either a structural problem, such as scarring on the pelvic organs, or a hormonal problem. Women will also be asked a great deal about their lifestyle, diet, and weight history. Presuming no other disorders, ovulation irregularities are usually caused by one of three things: excessive weight loss or weight gain, excessive exercise, and emotional stress (see chapters 2 and 3).

No competent infertility specialist will proceed with the workup without taking a full menstrual and contraceptive history. The doctor will be looking for a history of intrauterine device (IUD) usege as well as any signs of endometriosis or pelvic inflammatory disease (PID). The specialist will also make sure that you've been having regular menstrual cycles throughout the "trying to conceive" period for at least a year, that you've been timing your intercourse correctly, and that you've been having intercourse frequently during your ovulation peak. At this point, he or she should ask to see your BBT chart. (If you haven't been keeping a BBT chart, you'll need to start one and keep track of your cycles for at least three months. You won't see the specialist again until you have completed the charts.)

"What's the first test?" This question will have different answers depending on what your ovulation charts and medical history revealed. For an average woman who had no history of STDs, and had charts revealing normal patterns of ovulation, her specialist would most likely start with a post-coital test, proceed to an hysterosalpingogram, and finally to an endometrial biopsy. If a structural problem was suspected, some specialists may *immediately* check out the fallopian tubes before doing other tests, while others may still begin with the least invasive tests first, and gradually progress to the more invasive procedures. For the purposes of this chapter, I'll follow the "least invasive first" plan. Keep in mind that workup philosophy isn't necessarily better or worse, but simply a different *approach*. Finally, age does play a major role; the older you are, the speedier your workup needs to be. For a woman of average age (late 20s/early 30s), a workup should not last longer than a couple of months. If your workup is dragging on for more than three months, it's time to question your specialist.

As in the male workup, the female workup begins with a full physical: a pelvic exam, screening for STDs, Pap smear, blood work, and so on. If all goes well, you'll move on to the tests discussed throughout this chapter.

Sleuthing Out a Female-Factor Problem

Because the initial interview will set the stage for your workup, there are several clues your doctor will be on the lookout for:

- *Late menarche (having your first period after 18).* This is a sign that you may have a hormone imbalance.
- *Spotting between periods.* This could be a sign that your have a uterine abnormality of some sort.
- *Severe pelvic pain or cramping during menstruation (dysmenorrhea).* This could be a sign of endometriosis.
- *A "heavy" feeling in your pelvis.* This could mean you have a large fibroid. Treatment for fibroids is discussed in chapter 6.
- *History of abdominal or pelvic surgery.* Even if your surgery was unrelated to a gynecological problem (such as an appendectomy or bowel repair), scarring from the surgery could still affect your ovaries. Surgeries such as cesarean sections, removal of ovarian cysts, previous ectopic pregnancies, dilation and curretage (D & C), or abortion could definitely cause pelvic adhesions and scar tissue that may be obstructing your reproductive organs.
- *History of abnormal Pap smears.* If you were ever treated for an abnormal Pap with cone biopsies, laser surgery, or cryosurgery, these procedures can interfere with your cervical mucus.

Any surgery on your cervix could weaken it and may lead to an incompetent cervix, which will need to be stitched in the event of a pregnancy.

- *History of STDs.* You know this one. Again, chlamydia and gonorrhea can spell PID.
- *History of IUDs.* This device can predispose you to PID as well as an ectopic pregnancy.
- *Vaginal infections.* Any vaginal infection, such as yeast or "trich," can be toxic to sperm. It will be a "treat and repeat" situation.
- *Exposure to DES:* Are you a DES daughter?

The Pelvic Ultrasound

One of the least invasive procedures, a pelvic ultrasound is an excellent way for your doctor to get an idea of the size, shape, and dimensions of your pelvic organs. An ultrasound will also reveal whether your ovaries are producing follicles, and whether you have any unusual enlargements or inflammations that warrant specific tests. An ultrasound will also show whether your uterus is thickening accordingly, showing that you're making *enough progesterone,* which is crucial if the embryo is to implant itself in the uterus. The idea is to make sure that you don't have any obvious gynecological problems, or infections at work.

There are two methods of doing a pelvic ultrasound: transvaginally and abdominally. In Canada, most doctors will want to do both for insurance purposes.

Abdominal ultrasound

Abdominal ultrasounds require a full bladder, and many women will find it an uncomfortable procedure as a result. There are ways around the discomfort. You'll be given specific instructions to drink a large quantity of water (usually about eight glasses one hour prior to the procedure). For most women, this is just too much water! Before you begin drinking, call your clinic or doctor's office and find out whether you'll be seen *on time.* If the clinic is running behind, time your drinking accordingly. If you find that you're feeling uncomfortable before you even leave for your appointment, *empty your bladder completely.* By the time you arrive at the clinic and are called in to see the doctor, your bladder will have filled up again. If you arrive at the clinic and are in pain, ask for a paper cup and empty your bladder enough to fill it about 75%. This should tide you over. Finally, if you know that your bladder fills up quickly, all you need to do is drink half the water you're told to, or even one mug of coffee. That should be enough to fill your bladder for the appointment without causing extreme discomfort.

Ultrasound is also called *ultrasonography*. It is the use of an echo sounder to produce a picture of the pelvic tract. High-frequency, low-energy sound waves are used to scan your abdomen, reflecting your pelvis's outline on an electronic screen through a series of bright dots. A full bladder causes the uterus (normally lying behind the pelvic bones) to be pushed outward. This makes your reproductive organs easier to find and see on the scan. Jelly is rubbed all over your abdomen, and a probe (called a transducer) is placed on the jellied area and moved around. A computer translates the sound echoes into video pictures. This picture is called a *sonogram*. The operator will point out what the patterns in the video picture mean and will probably show you your parts on the screen. The procedure takes about ten minutes.

Since the ultrasound technologist does many ultrasounds in a day, you should make a point of telling him or her that you're there to investigate infertilty. This will tell the operator to take special note of unusual enlargements, cysts, scarring, fluid, and so on. Request a copy of the lab results from your doctor so you can discuss terminology and "normal variances" that may not seem so normal to *you*! For example, if you have a retroflexed uterus (tipped backward), your doctor may not bother to tell you about it (1 in 5 women do). Some doctors believe it's more difficult to conceive with this shape. If you have fluid in your cul-de-sac (the pocket surrounding your reproductive organs), your doctor may not find this significant, but you may want to know why the fluid is present. It may be an early indication of endometriosis.

Transvaginal ultrasound

You don't need to have a full bladder for this procedure, and some women prefer it to the abdominal procedure. At any rate, a transvaginal procedure can detect more than the abdominal ultrasound. A dildo-shaped transducer, with a condom over it and lubricated with jelly, is inserted into your vagina. If you can have comfortable intercourse, you shouldn't feel any pain at all. The procedure is usually performed by a female technician or supervised by a female. If you are very modest, you may request to insert the transducer yourself, but you must have very clean hands to avoid transferring bacteria. The procedure takes about ten minutes. Again, make sure you tell the technician why you're there so he or she can keep an eye open for red flags. Request a copy of the lab results from your doctor.

Testing for a Hormonal Problem

If your ultrasound results are normal, you'll begin a series of hormone tests that will be taken at different times in your cycle. The process begins by discussing your menstrual charts with your doctor, who may have observed some unusual patterns in the cycle right off the bat. For example, some BBT charts have flat patterns, whereas others have too many peaks and valleys.

Again, roughly 30% of all female infertility is caused by a hormonal imbalance of some sort. Depending on what kind of imbalance you have, you'll be plagued with different symptoms that include irregular cycles, failure of the embryo to implant in the uterus, poor-quality cervical mucus, or the inability to sustain a pregnancy, causing you to repeatedly miscarry (see chapter 9). Some ovulatory problems are not obvious. For example, even though you may not be ovulating every month, you could still have regular periods. This is known as an *anovulatory cycle*.

Blood Tests

When irregular ovulation is cited as the probable culprit, you'll undergo a series of simple blood tests done at various points in your cycle (different hormones peak at different times) to find what hormone is either missing, deficient, or exploding from your body. Assuming a 28-day cycle, on day 2 or 3 of your cycle, FSH, LH, and estradiol (a type of estrogen) are measured. Then, during the luteal phase (anywhere from days 22 to 24), progesterone levels are measured. Your doctor will check your levels of gonadotropin-releasing hormone (GnRH) and androgen levels. Prolactin levels can be checked at any time during your cycle, but it's best to do it in the morning, and for you to avoid touching your breast prior to the test. Touching your nipples or breasts, for example, may stimulate the hormone, and throw off the test, causing inaccurate results. You'll most likely undergo an(other) transvaginal ultrasound and endometrial biopsy (see further below) to accompany some of these blood tests.

Progesterone withdrawal test

This is an important test for women who have either bouts of *amenorrhea* (no periods) or chronic amenorrhea. This test determines whether the amenorrhea is caused by a uterine abnormality or a hormonal imbalance. Is the uterine lining getting thick enough to shed to begin with? If it isn't, you don't have the right amounts or combinations of hormones in your body to trigger a period. Is your uterus thickening each month but somehow not responding to your hormones, which is a signal to shed? There's an easy way to find out. Progesterone is given to you either orally or by injection to induce a period or "withdrawal bleeding." If the bleeding starts, then the problem is clearly a *hormonal* one. The hormonal problem will then need to be pinpointed by further tests. If you still do not bleed despite hormonal supplements there's either a *uterine* abnormality at work that will need to be ruled out, or you may not have enough estrogen to respond to the progesterone withdrawl.

If you have excessive body hair . . .

During your initial physical exam, your doctor will be checking to see if you have body hair on your breasts, back, abdomen, face, and so on. Your doctor may not notice that you have excessive hair because you might be *removing* it. If you're asked this question, you should answer truthfully. There is a condition known as *polycystic ovarian (PCO) syndrome*. This is a condition where your ovaries have small cysts that interfere with ovulation and hormone production. You'll also be asked about any skin problems such as acne, and you may also have a history of irregular periods and/or a battle with obesity. Obesity, oily skin and acne, irregular cycles, infertility, and excessive hair growth are symptoms of PCO.

If you have this problem, you're probably not ovulating regularly, which will show up in your menstrual charting. Your doctor will do some additional blood tests in this case to check for any elevated levels of *androgen*, a male hormone all women secrete in small amounts. You can also have elevated androgen levels and *not* have PCO. If androgen is the problem, you may need to be put on female hormone supplements such as estrogen replacement to offset it. PCO is treated with fertility drugs and is a classic, "textbook" cause of female infertility. See chapter 6 for more details.

If you're anovulatory, under five feet tall and suffer from a variety of chronic medical problems...

There is a genetic condition known as *Turner's syndrome*, which affects roughly 1 in 2500 women. Turner's women have either a missing or a damaged X chromosome (normally, women have two X chromosomes). These women are short, not growing beyond about 4'7", and usually have other medical problems, including ear, eye, heart, kidney, or thyroid disorders, diabetes, high blood pressure, and keloid healing.

These women also lack many secondary sexual characteristics (such as breasts or pubic hair), have irregular or nonexistent menstrual cycles, and are usually infertile. Other physical features include low-set ears, a low hairline, a webbed neck, pigmented moles, bending out of the elbows, and puffy hands and feet. Finally, while Turner's women are not mentally impaired and have the same IQ levels as the general population, many will suffer from learning disorders involving arithmetic and spatial skills (map reading, puzzles, visual problem-solving). Children with this problem may also be hyperactive.

If you suspect you have Turner's syndrome, request a *karotype study*, or a genetic test (via blood test), from your doctor. Fertility drugs will successfully treat Turner's and may alleviate other medical problems associated with it.

Cushing's syndrome

There is another disorder you can be tested for, known as *Cushing's syndrome*, which is an abnormality of the adrenal gland. Symptoms include irregular menstrual cycles or no menstrual cycles, a distinctive hump of fat between the shoulder blades, water retention (a.k.a. edema), high blood pressure, obesity, general muscular weakness, and easy bruising. Other characteristics include a moon-shaped face, acne, and abnormal hair growth (similar to PCO). Treating Cushing's syndrome is fairly simple. A steroid medication will return hormone levels to normal, which will reverse your infertility.

The Monitored Cycle

Some fertility specialists may want to place a woman on what's called a monitored cycle. If blood tests seem to be inconclusive, your doctor may want you to deliver a blood sample each day of your cycle, beginning on day 1. This way, he or she can get a clear picture of which hormones are appearing and disappearing within specific time frames of the cycle. A monitored cycle may also involve ultrasound, which can help establish whether you're developing follicles or whether your uterine is thickening accordingly.

This is an involved process that requires daily trips to a lab or the doctor's office, but the information it yields could nail down a hormonal imbalance. For example, one of the most difficult hormonal problems to diagnose has to do with *luteal phase defects*, discussed later in this chapter.

Monitored cycles are also done once you enter treatment, so your doctor knows exactly when you're ovulating for certain procedures such as IVF, IUI, or GIFT.

The Endometrial Biopsy

This is an in-office procedure that involves placing a small plastic cylinder inside the cervix. The cylinder contains a suction device that sucks up only a small portion of the endometrial lining.

The lining is then sent to a lab and analyzed. The procedure is an excellent diagnostic tool but is invasive and can be painful. Taking anti-inflammatory medication prior to the procedure will help take the edge off any cramping.

This biopsy procedure is used to investigate hormonal imbalances that can cause irregular cycles or annovulatory cycles, repeated miscarriages (see chapter 9), or even irregular uterine bleeding. It takes less than ten minutes to do and is far less invasive than a laparoscopic procedure.

For an infertility investigation, an endometrial biopsy is usually done between days 22-24 of the menstrual cycle (assuming a 28-day cycle). At the beginning of that cycle, your doctor will explain the importance of preventing pregnancy for that month. Abstinence or condoms are highly recommended during this interval. Prior to the biopsy, if you have any reason to suspect you're pregnant, a pregnancy test must be done to rule it out.

The purpose of the biopsy is to examine the characteristics of your endometrium to make sure it's the right consistency and thickness for that time of the month, which will indicate whether you're secreting the right *combination and levels* of hormones. Some doctors may choose to do the biopsy within the first 18 hours of your period, but this is trickier to time and to do. The outcome of your endometrial biopsy will determine whether you have a progesterone deficiency, an estrogen deficiency, or even an luteinizing hormone (LH) deficiency. Depending on the hormonal imbalance, you may just need a hormone supplement.

Prior to taking the test, your doctor will want you to keep a basal body temperature chart during the cycle of test, and perhaps for one cycle following. This will help him or her to put the results into context. You will also have your progesterone levels taken via blood test on the day of the test.

After the test, you can expect some cramping and spotting. Make sure you don't go home alone in case you have a bad time of it.

Few women will escape an endometrial biopsy during a female workup. This is a very important test that helps to pinpoint hormonal problems that may be suspected through a combination of blood tests, monitored cycles, and charting. While some of you may be recommended for treatment prior to the endometrial biopsy, most doctors will wait for the outcome of this test before recommending treatment.

Common Hormonal Problems

The results of all of the above tests will probably uncover one of the following hormonal disorders (unless you have PCO, Turner's syndrome, or Cushing's syndrome).

Post-oral contraceptive syndrome (a.k.a. post-pill syndrome)

It usually takes 3–12 months for your cycles to return to normal after going off oral contraceptives (OCs). Roughly 5% of the women who stop using OCs will not see normal cycles for over a year.

In these cases, fertility drugs may be suggested as well. Women who are prone to this usually had irregular cycles prior to taking their OC. It's crucial to note, however, that OCs do not *cause* infertility; they simply aggravate a preexisting fertility problem. Some of these women may also have hyperprolactinemia.

Hyperprolactinemia

Fifteen to 25% of irregular ovulation is caused by secreting too much of the hormone *prolactin*, which interferes with both ovulation and embryo implantation in the uterus.

Prolactin is released from the pituitary gland and is responsible for breast milk production. When levels are high, prolactin stops the pulsing of GnRH from the hypothalamus, which interferes with the pituitary gland's release of FSH and LH, interfering with estrogen and progesterone.

Normally, prolactin levels should be high only if you're pregnant or nursing. Otherwise, high levels can be caused by emotional or physical stress, exercise, nipple stimulation, or large intakes of protein (don't get your prolactin levels tested after you've eaten a giant steak!). Surgery around the rib cage can also raise prolactin levels. Drugs such as amphetamines, tranquilizers, antidepressants, hallucinogens, and alcohol may also be the culprit. If you have either PCO or an underactive thyroid gland (hypothyroidism), you can also have hyperprolactinemia.

Thirty percent of the time, women who have too much prolactin will notice milk in their breasts (called *galactorrhea)* or will notice milk when they squeeze their nipples during a breast self-exam. Other symptoms might include decreased vaginal secretions and irregular cycles. A woman may also have light, irregular, short, or no periods.

Hyperprolactinemia can be detected by a simple blood test. At least two blood tests will show high levels of prolactin. If the problem is caused by food, you may need to fast before retesting. Often these blood tests are followed up by a CAT scan to check for a possible *benign* pituitary tumor (occurring in about 5% of all women who have hyperprolactinemia). In fact, with chronically high levels of prolactin, a benign pituitary tumor known as a microadenoma (small) or a macroadenoma (large) is often the cause.

The drug bromocriptine (see chapter 7) usually offsets prolactin secretion and shrinks any tumors that exist. If a tumor is found, it can be surgically removed through the nasal passage, but this procedure may not restore your fertility. Radiation may also be used to shrink a pituitary tumor, but its rare in this case.

Premature ovarian failure

Premature ovarian failure is when your body goes into premature menopause. Your ovaries just "close shop." This is responsible for about 10% of all ovulation problems and, if you're under 30, your doctor may want to do a chromosome test. This is fairly easy to diagnose through blood tests and a pelvic exam. Some causes include a decreased number of eggs at birth (they get used up earlier), exposure to radiation or chemotherapy, chromosomal abnormalities, diseases such as cancer or AIDS, and physical trauma to the area (injuries and so on). Natural ovarian failure is diagnosed when you have very high levels of FSH and LH in your blood or urine, while your estrogen levels are very low.

This is not a treatable condition, but you may be put on hormone replacement therapy (HRT) to prevent osteoporosis and menopausal symptoms. In this situation, you and your partner have three choices: adoption, surrogate parenting, or childfree living. In some instances, if your uterus is still healthy, you can have an egg donated and try IVF using your partner's sperm. Premature ovarian failure is discussed more in chapter 6.

A deficiency in GnRH

GnRH triggers the release of FSH and LH from the pituitary gland. Without this, you won't ovulate. This is easily treated by replacing the hormone synthetically with fertility drugs. See chapter 7 for more details.

Luteal phase defects

This is when you don't have enough progesterone to keep your uterus embryo-friendly. Remember how the follicle bursts, and then turns into a corpus luteum, which secretes progesterone? Well, this stage of your cycle is also called the "luteal phase" and refers to a progesterone deficiency. Most women have a luteal phase that lasts 10–14 days. If your luteal phase lasts for less than 9 days or longer than 14 days, you may have a luteal phase defect. This is diagnosed from a blood test done during your luteal phase (the serum progesterone test) as well as an endometrial biopsy (see below). In this case, two endometrial biopsies are usually done to study variations on the lining's thickness in more detail. A third biopsy may be recommended if there is a question about the results. Your doctor will also look at your BBT chart and monitor your ovaries via ultrasound to try to catch your luteal phase (which will follow your follicular phase). You might want to review chapter 3 to recall how a normal cycle should work.

In a luteal phase defect, the corpus luteum stops working and doesn't produce enough progesterone to keep the endometrium thick enough for an embryo to implant itself. Luteal phase defects may also cause pregnancy loss if the embryo does implant, and is a common diagnosis in the event that you have more than two miscarriages. If you conceive with a luteal phase defect, usually the embryo is shed along with the endometrium lining (when you menstruate) before you would discover the pregnancy. This is known as an *occult pregnancy*.

In general, it's common for women to have luteal phase defects at some point during their menstrual lives. During puberty, around menarche (the first period), during the postpartum phase (after childbirth), and prior to menopause are when luteal phase defects strike the average woman. In these cases, the cycle usually corrects itself. Smoking and stress may also trigger this problem.

The diagnosis of a luteal phase defect has met with some controversy. Many U.K. researchers believe this luteal phase defect is incorrectly labeled; the reason why the corpus luteum is failing is because the follicle it originated from was a dud. In short, if the follicle was a "good egg" to begin with, the corpus luteum would not be failing. According to this line of thinking, if a good egg is produced during the *follicular phase* of the cycle, then all should go well in the second stage of the cycle. Many U.K. women will be treated with fertility drugs for this problem, in the belief that the drugs will help stimulate the ovaries to produce a *better* follicle, which in turn will develop into a better corpus luteum.

Most North American doctors, however, feel that treating a luteal phase defect with fertility drugs is akin to putting a bandage on a corpse. The feeling on this continent is that corpus luteum defects have nothing to do with how "good" the original egg is. Instead, the treatment recommended is to compensate for the failing corpus luteum by supplementing this phase of the cycle with progesterone. This will help to prime the endometrium during the luteal phase, making it more receptive to the embryo. These supplements will also help lower a woman's immune system response, preventing it from rejecting the embryo once it does implant. These supplements are given by vaginal or rectal suppository.

When you're taking a progesterone supplement, your doctor will need to monitor you via another endometrial biopsy to make sure that the supplements are working and that the dosage is correct. You'll need to be on these supplements for about four to five months before you can expect to conceive. In some cases, the supplements may continue during the first trimester of the pregnancy to reduce the chances of losing the pregnancy due to a lack of progesterone.

If the suppository doesn't work, the "British rules" for treatment are usually tried next. You'll be put on clomiphene citrate to see if your corpus luteum improves when your follicle production escalates. But clomiphene citrate, however, may *cause* luteal phase problems and even alter cervical mucus in ovulating women. In this case, intrauterine insemination can be done to compensate for the mucus problem. Some doctors will supplement either treatment (suppositories or fertility drugs) with an injection of human chorionic gonadotropin (HCG) within the third or fourth day of the luteal phase.

Hypothalamic amenorrhea

This is usually caused by a few of those seven habits discussed in chapter 2: weight loss, overexercise and stress, anorexia, and bulimia. An underactive hypothalamus or a late puberty may also trigger this problem. The symptoms include very light periods or no periods, and your blood tests will reveal very low hormones and no ovulation. You may have flat temperature readings and no mid-cycle cervical mucus.

If your lifestyle habits are the cause, your doctor will send you home and tell you to gain some weight, stop overexercising, try to relax, and so on. If this doesn't work, you will be probably be prescribed a regimen of hormonal supplements or fertility drugs. Even if you're planning on child-free living, women with constant low estrogen levels are at a high risk of developing osteoporosis.

Nonspecific anovulation (oligo-ovulation)

This means "we don't know why you're not ovulating." If you're ovulating less than 12 times a year and no cause for your irregular cycles are found, you'll be given this "diagnosis." The treatment is to put you on clomiphene citrate and wait. Pregnancy rates in this case are actually quite high.

You'll be relieved to know that ovulatory problems can almost always be treated with fertility drugs. This is known as *ovulation induction*. Between 60% and 90% of women treated for an ovulatory disorder go on to conceive. There *are* some drawbacks to fertility drugs, though. Women on clomiphene citrate, for example, may have problems producing high-quality cervical mucus and may not be able to sustain a pregnancy beyond the first trimester due to a luteal phase defect. All the drawbacks to fertility drugs are discussed in chapter 7. Pregnancy loss is discussed in chapter 9.

As a precaution, don't begin taking ANY fertility drugs before the cause of your ovulatory problems is nailed down. Some doctors tend to prescribe these drugs as soon as they see you're anovulatory, without bothering to find out WHY. In addition, just because you do have a hormonal imbalance doesn't mean there aren't other structural problems at work.

Testing Cervical Mucus

If you haven't yet read chapter 3, read the section on observing cervical mucus. While you may be ovulating right on schedule, you may not be producing high-quality cervical mucus. This is usually an indication that there is a hormonal problem at work, but the causes of poor cervical mucus are often unexplained. You should rule out infection before your doctor concludes that you're having mucus problems. Vaginal infections such as yeast or trich or other STDs will *absolutely* interfere with your cervical mucus production. Get this checked out if you haven't done so yet.

The Ferning or Spinbarkheit Test

The *ferning test* is so named because it involves drying a sample of your mid-cycle mucus to see if it forms a ferning pattern when it's examined under a microscope. Prior to ovulation (anywhere from days 10-15 of a 28-day cycle) as discussed in chapter 3, high-quality cervical mucus changes texture to a clear, stringy, and plentiful discharge that is very stretchy. This eggwhite consistency is known as *spinbarkheit*. This test involves getting into the "Pap" position, while your doctor collects cervical mucus for the test. That's it. Fairly non-invasive. Bear in mind that spinbarkheit refers to the stretchiness of the mucus when it's grasped with surgical instruments, such as clamps or forceps. The ferning test is usually done at the same time as the Postcoital Test, discussed next.

The Postcoital Test (PCT): Are You "Sperm-friendly?"

This is a simple, non-invasive test that is often one of the first tests performed during a female workup. Before going ahead with the PCT, some doctors may suggest that you use an LH test kit (see chapter 3), or may want you to undergo an ultrasound, which can help pinpoint ovulation. The postcoital test is far less invasive than a hysterosalpingogram. This test is painless but may be embarrassing. You'll need to make an appointment with your gynecologist around your mucus peak day. Then, you and your partner will need to have intercourse about 12 hours before the appointment (some doctors do it 2–4 hours after, but this isn't the best time). The timing depends on your schedule and the doctor's. When you arrive at your doctor's office, he of she will get you into the Pap position, and then insert a syringe high inside your vagina to collect your postcoital mucus. The doctor will also insert an instrument into your cervical canal to retrieve mucus. Your cervical opening should also be dilated slightly and will change in color around ovulation. Your doctor will make sure to check for this. The dilated opening allows more sperm through.

This is an important test, because it not only reveals the *relationship* between your partner's sperm and your cervical mucus, but it tells the doctor how well they're "getting along." The test also tells the doctor about your ovulation cycle. After collecting the postcoital mucus, your doctor places it under a microscope and examines it. The first thing that's checked is the cervical mucus consistency. It should be egg-whitelike, transparent, stretchy (stretching about 6–10 centimeters), have an alkaline pH balance (to match the pH balance of healthy sperm), be rich in mucin, glycoprotein and salt. If your mucus is too dry or scanty, or lacks these properties, the sperm will not be able to survive long enough to fertilize the ovum. The doctor will also check for sperm life signs, and the number of sperm present. *This is why 12 hours after intercourse is the best time for the test.* Since healthy sperm should be able to survive for *at least* 24 hours after intercourse, if there are no live sperm after 12 hours, there's a problem. The absence of sperm, or the presense of immobilized (live but paralyzed) sperm after 12 hours indicates that the mucus is rich in sperm antibodies, that sperm production is faulty—which would be an odd thing to discover after two *normal* semen analyses—or that intercourse positions are poor (ejaculating outside the vagina, or the penis is not placed high enough inside). Another reason why this test is best performed 12 hours after intercourse is because it puts far less pressure on the two of you. You can simply have intercourse the night before. This timing is preferable to some mad-dash interlude in the back seat of your car at lunch hour, and then racing to the doctor's office afterward.

If the test results are normal, you'll move on to the next stop: hysterosalpingogram.

What do the PCT results mean?

Roughly 15% of all female infertility problems *are* caused by poor-quality cervical mucus. If *this* is what the postcoital test finds, you may be put on estrogen supplements about 7–10 days before ovulation to try to raise the quality of the mucus. This doesn't work too often, though. A somewhat odd remedy that *has* been known to work, is taking *decongestant cough syrup* during the first two weeks of your cycle to increase mucus production throughout the body! In fact, this is considered the "answer" to infertility in some small towns. Some women have reported an increase in the quality and quantity of their mucus by using this method and *have* gotten pregnant as a result. (Sometimes truth really is stranger than fiction.) However, there is no definitive scientific evidence to support the cough syrup cure. In any event, many specialists will tell you to give it a try because this peculiar practice is harmless. You'll be asked to repeat the PCT a few times during your mucus Total Quality Management effort. If estrogen and cough syrups fail, the only other choice left to you is to have your partner's sperm placed high inside your uterus. This is known as *artificial insemination by husband* (AIH) (although your partner, of course, doesn't have to be your husband), or *intrauterine insemination* (IUI) with washed sperm.

If the PCT results find that the sperm are immobilized or dead, yet the semen analyses and cervical mucus are normal, your infertility may be caused by the presence of antisperm antibodies, known as *immunological infertility*, where your immune system manufactures antibodies that destroy your partner's sperm. This is also discussed in chapters 2, 4, and 6. Or, your intercourse position may have simply been a dud. With this kind of test result, you'll be asked to repeat the test. If you still get the same PCT result, immunological infertility is probably what's going on. This can be confirmed with further blood tests for both of you. There is no known effective treatment for this form of immunological infertility. Some doctors suggest clearing out all sperm from your system, wearing a condom for the next six months, and then trying again. The theory is that your body may relax once it's rid of it's "invader." Then, you can sneak the sperm back during ovulation and hopefully become pregnant before your immune system has time to destroy the sperm. Another theory is to put you on cortisone treatments to suppress your immune system; this has a very low success rate of about 25%. Otherwise, your only choice is IVF, discussed in chapter 8. Treating male-produced antisperm antibodies is discussed in chapter 6.

Making the most of your PCT

As mentioned above, you must have this test done prior to ovulation (around your mucus peak day). In order for there to be ample numbers of sperm, it's advised that your partner refrain from ejaculation 48 hours prior to having intercourse with you. When you have intercourse, you should refrain from using any lubricants or creams, which will interfere with the test results. Some doctors may want you to refrain from urinating prior to the the test, but this is an unreasonable demand if you're seeing the doctor several hours after intercourse. Some doctors suggest you remain still after intercourse for roughly 15 minutes to avoid losing any ejaculate, but again, this "holding-the-sperm-in" theory is highly controversial and dismissed as rubbish by most experts.

The PCT Cup Test

If the results from either your first or second PCT were ambiguous, your doctor may progress to the highly controversial PCT cup. Your partner delivers a semen sample while your cervical mucus is collected. Then, a small portion of both samples are placed on a glass side to see what happens. If the sperm penetrates the mucus, the rest of the semen is put into a plastic cup and placed over your cervix for about two hours (you can move around normally during this period). After two hours, *another* sample of mucus is collected, and survival rate of the sperm is assessed. Whether or not this test reveals anything terribly significant is in debate.

Penetrak Test (a.k.a. Bovine cervical mucus test)

This test crosses back into the male workup domain, but the results could pinpoint whether the problem is your mucus or his sperm, or a little bit of both. If the PCT result showed that the sperm had trouble penetrating your cervical mucus, the sperm may be placed inside thin tubes with cervical mucus from cows. The sperm is given about 90 minutes with the cows' mucus to see if the sperm can penetrate it. If the sperm react the same way to this mucus as they did to yours, then the problem is with the sperm. If, however, the sperm react differently to the cows' mucus than to yours, then the problem is truly with your cervical mucus and not his sperm.

Checking for Structural Problems

This is where the workup gets quite invasive. The procedures below may cause cramping and discomfort for a few hours. You'll need to arrange for appropriate time off when you have these procedures done. In other words, immediately heading to work after these tests isn't a good idea. Many specialists will perform the following tests in the late afternoon (3–5 P.M.) so you can return to work the next morning.

Looking into the Tubes: Hysterosalpingogram (HSG)

If your ovulation cycle is normal and you've passed your PCT with flying colors, it's time to check out the fallopian tubes. Basically, this test checks for symptoms of *salpingitis* and other signs of inflamed fallopian tubes caused by chlamydia or gonorrhea (see chapter 1), scarring from *endometriosis* (discussed in chapter 6), or scarring from past ectopic pregnancies. Your tubes can also become inflamed from previous abdominal surgery or a ruptured appendix. An HSG will also be done on women who want a tubal ligation reversed.

This test is invasive but quick. At best it's uncomfortable; at worst you'll feel *extremely* painful cramping. The pain *is* brief, however. Done in the first half of your cycle (after your period but prior to ovulation or days 7–11 of a 28-day cycle), you'll get into a Pap position, and your doctor will place a clamp on your cervix, which is uncomfortable. Your doctor injects a dye into the uterus, which should fly through your tubes and come out the other end. X rays are taken as the dye is injected and can detect whether the dye passes through the tubes' open ends or not. If the dye passes through, your tubes are open; if it doesn't, your tubes are blocked, which will make the test more painful.

Because this dye is a foreign substance, to prevent any risk of infection you may need to take antibiotics for about three days before undergoing this test. However, this is only done if you have a high risk of developing an infection. In addition, an allergy to iodine should be checked out prior to undergoing the test. Some doctors recommend that you take anti-inflammatory medication prior to the test to reduce cramping. Even if your tubes are open, the dye can cause discomfort. It will be expelled as a sticky discharge from the vagina, and the rest will be absorbed by your body.

What do the results show?

This test can be inconclusive. For example, if the dye flows through your tubes freely, you may *still* have a problem with the quality of your *cilia* (small hairs that line our tubes and cavities). This may prevent smooth delivery of the egg through the tube into the uterus.

The test may not be successful in picking up pelvic adhesions, endometriosis, or problems with the *fimbria* (fringes at the ends of the tubes). It will usually pick up abnormalities affecting the tubal block or uterine structures, endometrial polyps, fibroids, and adhesions in the uterus itself.

Are there any risks?

The HSG can cause pelvic inflammatory disease (PID) by carrying bacteria into your tubes. Because of this, you should be given antibiotics prior to the test. If your tubes are blocked, your doctor may want to do a laparoscopy (see below). Or, he or she may suspect PID and treat you with an aggressive antibiotic regimen (see chapter 6). Laparoscopy will also find other structural problems caused by PID, cysts, or endometriosis. Repair surgery is discussed in chapter 6.

Laparoscopy

Laparoscopy is the most invasive test of all, but you won't feel it because you'll be under a general anesthetic. This test is usually considered the last one done in a female workup. If, however, your doctor strongly suspects endometriosis, this may be one of the first procedures you undergo. The only way to absolutely diagnose endometriosis is through a laparoscopy.

For this test, you'll need to check into a hospital as a day patient. Under a general anasthetic, a long thin tube, called a *laparoscope*, is inserted into your abdominal cavity. This cavity is inflated with carbon dioxide so the walls are forced away from the organs so that the doctor can get a good look inside your abdominal and pelvic cavity. Light from a projector outside the tube is passed through the cables containing hollow glass wires. The surgeon can now get a clear, three-dimensional view of your ovaries, fallopian tubes, uterus and peritoneum (pelvis lining), gall bladder, spleen and liver, and large and small intestines.

Sometimes referred to as "keyhole surgery," the laparoscope is inserted into your abdomen through a tiny incision in the belly button. Sometimes a second small incision is made above the pubic bone, and a thin probe is inserted to help move organs around.

A more in-depth HSG may be done at this point, as a blue dye is passed through your fallopian tubes, giving your doctor a better idea of the condition of the tubes. In addition, some minor corrective procedures may be done, such as burning away spots caused by endometriosis. Your surgeon may also do a hysteroscopy. Here, a device is inserted directly into your uterus, which will hunt for tumors, adhesions, and congenital abnormalities. Finally, a tuboscopy may be done as well, in which a scope is put right inside your fallopian tube to examine its lining.

The laparoscopy takes about 20–30 minutes. After the procedure, the carbon dioxide gas will slowly escape through the incision prior to stitching. You may feel discomfort in your chest or shoulders if not all of the gas was released. Don't worry about this. The gas will eventually be absorbed. A laparoscopy reveals nothing unusual 50% of the time. If you have any tumors, cysts, endometriosis, pelvic adhesions, or scarring, laparoscopy will find it. Most women need to be off work for a few days after the procedure. You may have a bad reaction to the anesthetic and need to rest. You may also feel nauseated and tired for a couple of days following the procedure. You should expect some cramping and mild abdominal discomfort; however, many women find they have no symptoms and can return to work the day after surgery.

If you're experiencing extreme discomfort and pain and/or have a fever, report this to your doctor immediately. You may have contracted an infection.

What's the Next Step?

For most couples, a female workup will finally reveal the cause of your infertility. For others, it may reveal that a female factor problem exists *along* with a male-factor problem (discovered in the event that treatment is sought out for a male-factor problem). Or, the infertility may be unexplained. Whatever the results are, you will need to move on to the next part of the fertility journey: treatment. Fertility drugs can usually treat any hormonal problems that exist for a female factor problem. However, when the problem is structural, many microsurgical techniques have poor results and may not increase your chances of conceiving. Under these circumstances, it's important to truly educate yourself about your options, the costs, the time involved in treatment, and the emotional investment you'll need to make. All of these issues are discussed in chapters 6, 7, and 8.

Unexplained Infertility

Ten to 15% of couples will not find an identifiable cause for their infertility. Of those, 20% will get pregnant each year for three years. It may be a relief that nothing is "technically" wrong with you, but it's also a maddening predicament. The situation can create tension in your relationship and may be aggravated by rude or tactless remarks from outsiders.

Just because your infertility is unexplained doesn't mean you cannot seek out treatment. Fertility drugs and a number of ART procedures can be ideal solutions to this problem. See chapters 7 and 8 for more details.

Refusal of Treatment

Some of you may not want to go beyond this point. You may have discovered a problem that isn't treatable, or you may have discovered that a female factor problem exists along with a male factor problem. You may have unexplained infertility, or you may have a treatable problem, but you may not *want* to be treated.

For many people, the idea of not treating a fertility problem seems incomprehensible. How could you not want to *fix* the problem? Remember that just because a problem *is* treatable, there is no guarantee that you'll conceive. For some, the idea of refusing treatment is an ideal option.

Treatment involves repeating various aspects of both the male and female workup, investing a great deal of time and energy (including time off work), and investing a great deal of money. Couples with limited financial resources may not be able to make the stretches and compromises that treatment demands. Other couples who are financially secure may just feel comfortable accepting what nature has in store: "If we get pregnant spontaneously, great. If we don't, that's fine too." Again, the next chapter may be in order or out of order, depending on what you decide.

6

What's the Problem
and How Do We Fix It?

In the previous two chapters, I discussed the diagnostic journey involved in finding either a male factor or female factor cause for your infertility. This chapter addresses the course of treatment for your infertility. For many of you, the buck stops here. Whether your problem is hormonal or structural, once the problem is fixed you may conceive without difficulty. For others, fixing the problem may not be that simple, and conception delays may persist. Under these circumstances, you may need to move on to further treatments involving assisted reproductive technology (ART), discussed in chapter 8.

For many female fertility problems, treatment entails fertility drugs such as clomiphene citrate (Clomid, Serophene), human menopausal gonadotropin (Pergonal or Metrodin), and several others. These drugs are powerful and potent. Some women will experience side effects, and some may be reluctant to use fertility drugs because of studies that suggest a link between them and ovarian cancer. Some men may also be placed on fertility drugs if their fertility is linked to a hormonal problem. Chapter 7 covers fertility drugs in detail.

Female Factor Infertility

Roughly 30% of all female factor infertility is caused by hormonal problems. Common hormonal disorders revealed by the female workup (see chapter 5) can be treated with fertility drugs or hormone supplements. Polycystic ovarian syndrome, a more complicated hormone disorder, carries a variety of treatment options. Ovarian failure, another disorder, is a consequence of many cancer therapies as well as exposure to certain environmental toxins. Both are discussed below.

The remaining 50–60% of all female factor infertility is caused by a structural problem, and pelvic inflammatory disease (PID) or endometriosis is usually the culprit. Both conditions, along with less common structural problems, are below as well.

Polycystic Ovarian Syndrome (a.k.a. Polycystic Ovarian Disease or Stein-Leventhal Syndrome)

Polycystic ovarian syndrome (PCO) is a classic female infertility problem. About 4% of the general female population suffers from PCO, which accounts for half of all hormonal disorders affecting female fertility.

With PCO, your body secretes far too much androgen, which counteracts your ovaries' ability to make enough progesterone necessary for a normal cycle. Your estrogen levels are fine, though, and your levels of lutenizing hormone (LH) are higher than usual, working overtime to try to kick-start the cycle. But the androgen levels interfere with your follicle stimulating hormone (FSH), which you need to trigger progesterone. As a result, your follicles never develop, and instead turn into small, pea-size cysts on your ovaries. Your ovaries can then enlarge. The elevated androgen levels can also cause you to develop facial hair, hair on other parts of your body (this happens in 70% of the cases and is called *hirsutism*), or even a balding problem. Acne is another typical symptom, as well as obesity, although women who are thin or of normal weight can also have PCO. Your periods will be irregular, and as a result you might be at greater risk for developing *endometrial hyperplasia*, in which your uterine lining thickens to the point of becoming precancerous. (If you have endometrial hyperplasia, progesterone supplements will be given to you to induce a period, or a dilatation and curettage (D & C) may be done to eliminate the lining.) Because of your high levels of androgen, you may also be at an increased risk for cardiovascular disease. Diet can help reduce the onset of heart problems.

If PCO was caught early on in your menstrual history, you simply would have been put on combination oral contraceptives to induce normal withdrawal bleeding and pump your system with normal levels of estrogen and progesterone. Or you would have been put on progestin, a synthetic progesterone supplement, and would have been instructed to take it about mid-cycle.

If you were treated earlier with progestin, you won't experience problems with your cycle unless you go off the drug for some reason. But women who were treated with oral contraceptives for irregular cycles at a very young age may not know *why* they suffered from irregular periods to begin with (see chapter 3). When these women go off contraception to conceive, they will be plagued by the same symptoms that initially warranted oral contraception. Sometimes women with normal cycles may develop PCO later in life. In this case they will suddenly develop irregular cycles (called *secondary amenorrhea*).

Why are estrogen levels normal in PCO women?

Normal estrogen levels come as a surprise to women with PCO. In normally fertile women, estrogen is made from the follicles. In this case, however, your body converts the *androgen* into estrogen. If you're obese, estrogen will also be stored in fat cells. This constant estrogen level confuses the hypothalamus, which assumes that high estrogen levels are present because of a developing egg inside the follicle. The hypothalamus will then tell the pituitary to slow down the release of FSH. Without FSH, your follicles won't mature and burst and hence you won't ovulate.

Who's at risk for PCO?

PCO is hereditary and is more common among women of Mediterranean descent. It's also uncommon to develop PCO later in life, although it can happen. Generally, a PCO woman will begin to experience menstrual irregularities within 3–4 years after her menarche (first period). Women who are obese can be predisposed to PCO because their fatty tissues produce estrogen, which can confuse the pituitary gland. Women who are diabetic or who have a problem with their adrenal glands, thyroid gland, or pituitary gland can develop symptoms of PCO, but technically not have the condition. Make sure you ask your doctor to rule out these conditions before you begin any treatment for PCO. In some cases, PCO may coincide with these conditions.

Reversing infertility

To reverse infertility in women with PCO, doctors will use the fertility drug clomiphene citrate (Clomid or Serophene) in tablet form. You'll start clomiphene citrate on day 5 of your cycle, then go off the tablet on day 10. If you've had long bouts of amenorrhea, your period will be induced via a progesterone supplement before you start on clomiphene citrate. An average dosage of clomiphene citrate in this case ranges between 25 and 50 milligrams. In some cases, an anti-estrogen drug called *tamoxifen* (also used as treatment in certain kinds of breast and gynecological cancers) may also be used with clomiphene citrate. Roughly 70–90% of all PCO women on clomiphene citrate will ovulate, but pregnancy rates vary; 30–70% of PCO women on clomiphene will conceive.

If you're still not ovulating after taking clomiphene, human chorionic gonadotropin (HCG) may be added to your hormonal "diet" during the luteal phase of your cycle, roughly one week after your last dose of clomiphene citrate.

If this regimen fails, you'll graduate to Metrodin (human menopausal gonadotropin—HMG), which is a very potent fertility drug. This drug is *pure* FSH, made from the urine of menopausal women. (During menopause, FSH naturally soars in the body to compensate for tired ovaries.) Prior to starting Metrodin, you'll need to have an hysterosalpingogram (see chapter 5) to make sure that your fallopian tubes are clear. You may also need a pelvic ultrasound to rule out other structural abnormalities. PCO women don't fare as well on Metrodin as they do on clomiphene citrate. While 70–80% will ovulate with Metrodin, only 20–40% will conceive. While taking Metrodin, you'll also need to be monitored through blood tests (to check estrogen levels) and ultrasound (to check follicle growth). The side effects, costs, and risks associated with clomiphene citrate and Metrodin are discussed in chapter 7. Multiple births are also common with both drugs.

Other treatments for PCO

In many PCO women, weight loss is considered the "cure." However, when infertility is a concern and a PCO patient wants to conceive, weight loss is not really a realistic short-term treatment because it's a slow, time-consuming process. If you have PCO and are being treated with fertility drugs, you may be able to reverse your fertility through natural weight loss for future pregnancies. You'll need to see a nutritionist and design a weight loss program that's in tune with your lifestyle.

If the ovaries have large cysts on them, some fertility specialists may want to try to cauterize the ovary in about 8–10 small spots through laparoscopic surgery. Roughly 62% PCO women who undergo it successfully go on to conceive, and when the surgery is combined with fertility drug therapy, the pregnancy rates are as high as 80%.

In some PCO women, androgens are also produced in the adrenal glands. Under these circumstances, your doctor may want to put you on a corticosteroid to suppress the adrenal gland, lowering the production of androgens. This will help induce ovulation as well.

Bromocriptine (discussed in chapter 7), which suppresses prolactin, will be given to 15–20% of all PCO women. The high levels of estrogen associated with PCO commonly cause hyperprolactinemia (see chapter 5).

Treating hirsutism

Because one of the unpleasant symptoms of PCO is hirsutism, which results in excessive male-patterned hair growth on the face, navel, or breasts, many women will want treatment. An antiandrogen drug, which is available in pill or cream form, will take care of the hair growth problem. You'll need to discuss the exact dosage of this drug with your doctor. Hair growth should slow down after about five months on the drug.

In the interim, electrolysis is the most effective treatment for hair growth on the face, navel, or breasts. Make sure you go to a reputable clinic and ask to talk to past clients. Sloppy electrolysis can result in burning and other skin problems.

Premature Ovarian Failure

As discussed briefly in chapter 5, ovarian failure is when your ovaries shut down, resulting in a premature menopause. Depending on the degree of ovarian failure, ovulation induction may be attempted with fertility drugs. If this fails, there is no way to treat the condition, although hormone replacement therapy may be suggested to prevent *menopausal* symptoms. There are several options available to women at risk for this, however.

Who's at risk?

Any woman undergoing chemotherapy or radiation therapy to her abdominal or pelvic region is at risk for premature ovarian failure. Hodgkin's disease, non-Hodgkin's lymphoma, and leukemia are classic cancers that strike women in their teens and 20s. Breast cancer, rare in women under the age of 35, may result in infertility for women who have delayed having children until their mid-to-late 30s. Disturbing increases in a variety of skin cancers, such as melanoma, can strike women who overexpose themselves to the sun while they are still in their childbearing years. Keep in mind that not all chemotherapy treatments will result in ovarian failure. Dosages in some cases have been refined to the point where ovarian function resumes uninterrupted, although an early menopause (prior to age 40) is often the consequence.

Women exposed to occupational hazards, including chemicals and radiation, or to radiation from environmental fallout are also at risk for premature ovarian failure. See chapter 2 for more details.

In some cases, premature ovarian failure is due to natural causes (being born with a limited number of eggs), congenital abnormalities, and so on. If your mother went into an early menopause, you may be at risk for premature menopause yourself.

Options to maximize your fertility

No woman will undergo chemotherapy or radiation treatments without being informed about the risks to her fertility. Although in most cases the loss of fertility may be a secondary concern over the potential loss of one's life, there are a few options you can consider if you want to have a biological child. Depending on your situation, none of these options may be possible or feasible, but it doesn't hurt to ask.

- Discuss the idea of retrieving some of your eggs *prior* to your treatment. These eggs can be frozen and used later for an in vitro fertilization (IVF) or a gamete intrafallopian transfer (GIFT) procedure with your partner's sperm when you're well again. (You still may be able to carry a child if your uterus is intact and healthy.) You can also use these eggs in a "host uterus" of a surrogate mother who is impregnated with an embryo resulting from your egg and your partner's sperm. Bear in mind that this procedure is still in the experimental stage, though.

- If you're receiving external radiation therapy to your pelvic region, investigate whether an *oophoropexy* can help prevent ovarian failure. This is a surgical procedure that moves your ovaries out of the path of the radiation beam. Then, after the treatment, the ovaries are repositioned and your ovarian function can resume. If you're receiving chemotherapy either alone or in conjunction with radiation therapy to the pelvic region, an oophoropexy will be ineffective.

- There is a procedure known as an "ovary transplant". Here, your ovaries are removed and frozen prior to cancer therapy. Then, when you're well again, your own healthy ovaries are transplanted back into your body. Ask your doctor about whether you're a candidate for this.

- Discuss the risks of *delaying* your treatment for one year so you can get pregnant prior to your therapy.

- After treatment, get pregnant as soon as possible. You'll usually be cautioned to wait two years after chemotherapy before you can try to get pregnant. Depending on your dosage of chemotherapy, ovarian function may resume for a few years before menopause sets in. Try to get pregnant as soon as your doctor considers it safe. If you're not married and are not in a position to have a child yet, you may want to consider having your eggs retrieved and frozen for later use just in case ovarian function shuts down earlier.

Pelvic Inflammatory Disease (PID)

PID is a general term that refers to infection and inflammation of one or more of your pelvic organs: your cervix, uterus, fallopian tubes, or ovaries (known as your *upper genital tract*). These infections can also spread to other parts of your body, infecting your abdominal cavity, kidneys, liver, lungs, and so on. PID is a serious condition that affects well over one million women each year in North America. In the United States alone, about 300,000 women are hospitalized because of PID; 1,000 women die from PID annually, and over $4.2 billion is spent on treatment. This disease is also a major cause of female factor infertility in North America. Because of the availability of ultrasound and laparoscopy, PID is also a newly recognized disease that wasn't really diagnosed until the early 1970s. Prior to the 1970s, women with PID were often misdiagnosed or branded hypochondriacs when they complained of chronic pelvic pain or other PID symptoms.

What causes PID?

Bacteria is the cause of PID. Normally, the cervix acts as a barrier, preventing bacteria from getting inside the upper pelvic region. But when the uterus is invaded by a sexually transmitted disease (STD) or is dilated for any reason, bacteria can enter and do a lot of damage. For example, when certain bacterial STDs—primarily gonorrhea and chlamydia—remain untreated, the infection can spread and cause PID. Bacteria can also enter your pelvic region through intrauterine device (IUD) insertion, the second major cause of PID in countries that use IUDs. Douching, certain pelvic surgical procedures such as abortions, D & Cs, amniocentesis, or natural phenomena such as miscarriages and childbirth can also cause PID. Smoking increases a woman's risk of PID. Both current and past smokers were found to be twice as likely to develop the disease. The reasons why are *not* known, however. The irony is that in the majority of cases, PID is preventable.

Symptoms

Because PID is a general label that doesn't tell you where the infection is, the symptoms can vary depending on what organ is infected. Although there are several symptoms associated with PID, the common pattern is to experience only one or two of them. Some women have only mild symptoms, some women have symptoms so severe they can't function, and other women experience no symptoms at all and may discover they have PID only when they investigate infertility.

The most common symptom is lower abdominal pain. It may be sporadic or chronic and may occur only during or after intercourse, menstruation or ovulation. The pain is often on one side of the abdomen and increases with movement, such as walking or climbing. The pain is always present during a pelvic examination, when your doctor feels your pelvic region manually to check for enlargements or abnormalities. Sometimes the pain is present when you urinate or move your bowels.

Other symptoms include lower back pain, nausea and dizziness, a low fever, chills, bleeding between periods, bleeding after intercourse, heavier menstrual cramps and flows, frequent urination, burning during urination or an inability to empty the bladder, unusual vaginal discharge with a foul odor, constantly feeling like you have to move your bowels, a general feeling of ill health, and abdominal bloating.

It's most common for PID to localize in the fallopian tubes, causing *salpingitis*, or inflammation of the fallopian tubes. The tubes close up or scar as a result, which is why infertility is often the result (it's often reversible, however). Ectopic pregnancy can also result from PID for the same reasons. PID is divided into three categories of infection: *acute*, meaning severe; *subacute*, meaning less severe; and *chronic*, meaning that you have a fresh acute infection or that scarring has developed as a result of a previous infection.

Diagnosing PID

For many women undergoing a female workup, PID is suspected when an hysterosalpingogram reveals blocked tubes. However, prior to undergoing an hysterosalpingogram, PID can often be diagnosed during a normal pelvic exam. In this exam, your doctor should always perform what's known as a *bimanual examination*. Two fingers are inserted into your vagina, while your abdomen on the outside is felt with the other hand simultaneously. This procedure is comparable to fitting a comforter inside its cover: one hand on the inside, the other on the outside to adjust and feel for contours and abnormalities. Pain and swelling are classic signs of PID that an experienced gynecologist or primary care physician will notice immediately. Then, during the speculum examination, your doctor will look for pus that might be coming out of the cervix, a symptom of *cervicitis* (inflammation of the cervix). If your cervix is red or swollen for any reason, a Pap test might be done as well. If pus is found, a sample will be sent to a lab for analysis, and a vaginal swab will also be taken to look for bacteria. At this point, the bacteria causing your pain (and PID) might be identified right off the bat, and the appropriate antibiotic medication will be prescribed. You could conceivably be cured at this point. Your partner will also need to be treated to prevent reinfecting you or someone else.

A blood test can also indicate whether you're fighting an infection of some sort. If you are, you'll have increased levels of white blood cells and an elevated sedimentation rate. An ultrasound test is also helpful. It can show whether an abscess has developed on the fallopian tubes or ovaries.

Finally, if all else fails, a laparoscopy can be performed which will definitely confirm a PID diagnosis. A laparoscopy might also be done if the doctor suspects that you have abscesses (resulting from severe inflammation) which have burst, a potentially life-threatening situation.

Once your PID is diagnosed, successfully treating PID is dependent on identifying the right bacteria responsible for the infection in the first place, so you can be treated with the *right* antibiotic! This isn't always easy. There are three procedures used to obtain a culture of the PID bacteria. The first is obtaining a cervical culture. The second procedure is called a *culdocentesis*, similar to amniocentesis, where fluid is taken out of the cul-de-sac, an area in your pelvic cavity where fluid tends to collect. A long needle is used to withdraw the fluid, which is then sent to a lab. The procedure is done under a local anesthetic in a hospital. Another technique used is a *tubal sample*. Here, fluid and tissue samples from your fallopian tubes are obtained during a laparoscopy procedure and sent to a lab for bacterial analysis.

Antibiotic therapy: the PID treatment

The beauty of bacterial infections is that they can be destroyed with antibiotics. Antibiotic therapy is the most common treatment regimen for acute and subacute PID. Even chronic PID can be treated successfully with antibiotics. Since PID indicates such a serious infection, antibiotics are given intravenously as a therapy; they're more potent this way and work faster. When several different types of bacteria are identified in PID, this is known as a *polymicrobial* infection. If this is the case, you may either be treated with more than one kind of antibiotic simultaneously, or you might be treated with a single, broad-spectrum antibiotic, which is less effective.

By far the best treatment approach is intravenous antibiotic therapy. To receive intravenous antibiotics, you'll need to be admitted into the hospital for about four days, the usual treatment duration. Ten to 14 days of oral antibiotics may follow in conjunction with bed rest.

What are the recommended antibiotics?

There many different kinds of antibiotic regimens that work. The following is a sample regimen. For PID caused by gonorrhea and/or chlamydia, 100 milligrams of doxycycline by IV (intravenous) twice a day, plus 2 grams of cefoxitin (an antibiotic used to cure gonorrhea) four times a day by IV is the standard treatment for about four days, followed by 100 milligrams of doxycyline twice a day for about 14 days.

For PID caused by chlamydia and/or anaerobic bacteria (a certain strain of bacteria), treatment is 100 milligrams of doxycycline by IV, plus 1 gram of metronidazole twice a day for about four days, followed by the same dosages of both drugs orally twice a day for about 14 days.

For PID caused by anaerobic bacteria or facultative gram-negative rods (other strains of bacteria), 600 milligrams of clindamycin four times a day by IV, plus gentamicin or tobramycin at a dosage of 2 milligrams for each kilogram of body weight, followed by 1.5 milligrams per kilogram three times a day for four days, then 450 milligrams of clindamycin four times a day orally for about 14 days is the treatment.

If you're already pregnant but don't know it yet or if you have other health problems, other antibiotics will be recommended. The above antibiotics are prescription only, and these doses are generally recommended for women who aren't pregnant and who are otherwise healthy.

What are the side effects of these antibiotics?

Yeast infections are a main side effect, because antibiotics interrupt the vaginal ecosystem. However, each antibiotic carries individual side effects. *Doxycycline* can cause nausea, yeast infections, allergies, liver damage (particularly in pregnant women), and brown discoloration of teeth in children. *Cefoxitin* (fine for pregnant women but not always for women allergic to penicillin) can cause allergies and kidney damage. *Metronidazole* (Flagyl) results in nausea, headache, loss of appetite, metallic taste, dark urine, abdominal pain, constipation, inflammation of the tongue or mouth, yeast infections, and deposits in breast milk (*therefore unsafe for pregnant women*) and cannot be combined with alcohol. *Clindamycin* brings on diarrhea, colitis, allergies, temporary abnormalities in liver function.

What should I do after my antibiotic treatment?

Get rechecked by your doctor to make sure you are indeed cured. Request another bacterial culture to make sure it's been destroyed, and make sure your partner is treated for the same bacterial infection. Otherwise, you could be re-infected. You should also abstain from intercourse until you are pronounced cured. Intercourse can spread pus in your pelvic cavity while you're healing.

Reversing infertility

Most cases of reversing infertility from PID involve reopening the fallopian tubes. This is known as a *tuboplasty*. The surgery is delicate and is done through laparoscopy. If your PID is severe and your tubes are badly scarred, a tuboplasty may not be possible and you'll need to seek out ART options that do not require healthy fallopian tubes but can be done if your ovaries and uterus are intact. If your tubes are intact but scarring exists elsewhere, your scarring may be removed through laparoscopy. The one problem with having a tuboplasty or other pelvic repair surgery is that fresh scarring may result. The risk of ectopic pregancy can also increase. Because of this, a "second look" laparoscopy may be recommended, which is discussed toward the end of this section.

In some cases, PID results in abscesses that MUST be surgically removed before they burst and spread infection throughout your pelvis and upper abdominal region. This surgery would be performed as a life-preserving measure rather than a fertility repair procedure.

Surgical treatment for PID

Inflammation is one thing, abscesses are another. An abscess occurs when the inflamed tissue forms a collection of pus. The abscess can then rupture and spread the bacterial infection, causing your PID to infect other parts of your pelvic region. In many cases of PID, abscesses may not even develop. But when they do, surgical removal of the abscess may be necessary, and even surgical removal of the badly abscessed *organ* may be an option. In either case, surgery is either emergency or elective.

If your abscesses have ruptured or are about to rupture, your doctor will schedule emergency surgery. *Emergency surgery need not be major surgery* and can involve simply removing the adhesions through laparoscopy or even laparotomy, a procedure similar to laparoscopy, where a four-inch incision is made in the abdomen, resulting in very little scarring. However, it's crucial that you discuss exactly what *kind* of surgery to expect, and take every precaution to preserve your reproductive organs if possible. Both laparoscopy and laparotomy procedures are considered major surgery, and you'll be required to go under a general anesthetic. A laparotomy is also performed if a *salpingectomy*, surgical removal of the fallopian tubes, is necessary. Depending on the severity of your PID and the location of the infection, this might actually be the best option for you. As mentioned above, it's most common for PID to localize in the fallopian tubes, which can cause a host of uncomfortable and painful symptoms for you. If the tubes are badly infected and have abscessed, removing them may just be the answer.

Removing the tubes is often done to preserve your ovaries and uterus, preventing the PID from spreading further and facilitating ART techniques that do not involve the tubes. If abscesses have formed in the uterus or on the ovaries, more drastic surgery may be necessary in the form of either a hysterectomy or *oophorectomy* (surgical removal of the ovaries), or both.

If surgery is being recommended to relieve your pain but there are no active infections, abscesses, or inflammations present, a procedure known as a *presacral neurectomy* is an option. In this operation, the sensory messages from the organs of the pelvis, carried along the presacral nerve, are eliminated by removing the nerve itself. Hence, the pain is also eliminated. This is also major surgery and requires a very skilled surgeon, since the nerve is close to large blood vessels. It is also a more difficult operation to perform than a hysterectomy, but the surgery is about 75% effective in eliminating pelvic pain (a promising statistic) and does not affect fertility. One interesting side effect is that if a woman gets pregnant after the procedure, she will experience less pain during labor or childbirth! The procedure can interfere with bowel and bladder function (which usually clears up on its own). To what extent this procedure affects sexual sensations or even menstrual cramps has not yet been statistically tracked. A presacral neurectomy is considered a last resort for relieving pelvic pain associated with PID and is only a *palliative* solution, not a cure.

Prevention

The good news is that in almost all cases, *PID is a completely preventable disease*. The number-one cause of PID in North America is an untreated STD; chlamydia and gonorrhea are the two STDs that are considered "principally implicated" in causing PID. Translation: You can prevent STDs by practicing safe sex. Currently, vaccines for chlamydia and gonorrhea are being researched and may soon be introduced as standard vaccines available to the general public. In addition to choosing uninfected partners, postponing intercourse with new partners for as long as possible, and using barrier methods, notifying sex partners after discovering any STD is an important step in primary prevention. In fact, women are not considered cured of PID unless their partners are treated for the initial PID-causing STD as well. Partners of women with PID have infection rates as high as 53% for chlamydia and 41% for gonorrhea, and a large percentage of these infections are asymptomatic.

Another crucial step in preventing PID is educating yourself about the risks involved with certain contraceptives. It is an undisputed fact, for example, that women who use IUDs are *three to nine times* as likely to develop PID. Why? First, bacteria, normally screened by your cervix, can enter your uterus during IUD insertion. (Some experts counter that taking doxycycline prior to insertion will reduce the risk of infection.) Second, even if no bacteria enters during insertion, the IUD can irritate your uterus later on, causing a local infection.

As a rule, whenever your cervix is dilated for *any* reason (childbirth, miscarriage, D & C, abortion, IUD insertion), avoid getting *anything* into your vagina for about six weeks, or *until your cervix has closed up again*. This means no baths (showers are fine, though), no swimming, no intercourse, sex toys, douching, or tampons! See your doctor to make sure that the cervix has resumed its usual shape and appearance.

There is also evidence that hormonal contraceptives affecting your cervical mucus may increase your chances of contracting an STD during unprotected sex. Apparently, the mucus is not as effective in screening out harmful bacteria as "untampered," or natural mucus is.

Douching is also a factor in primary prevention. Douching may alter the vaginal environment and make it less protective against harmful bacteria, and douching might flush vaginal and cervical bacteria into the upper pelvic region, causing infections.

Finally, basic vaginal hygiene habits, discussed in chapter 2, in addition to good overall nutrition, can also help prevent PID. Even if you can't afford proper health insurance, you can improve your overall nutrition and hygiene regimen.

If you're not practicing safe sex, request a screening for chlamydia and gonorrhea before you have sex with a new partner.

If you notice any kind of unusual symptom that may indicate an STD, see your doctor and request a diagnosis or prompt antibiotic treatment for suspected STDs. Never self-diagnose! Treating an STD quickly will prevent it from causing PID.

Endometriosis

The first case of endometriosis was possibly documented in 1600 B.C., according to ancient Egyptian writings. However, endometriosis was not recognized as a real disease until the twentieth century. In the past, endometriosis either was considered rare or was simply undiagnosed; today, it's a major cause of painful periods and infertility in women.

In fact, the majority of women with endometriosis complain about pain, and until quite recently, a large percentage of them (one endometriosis clinic reports as many as 75%) were dismissed as neurotic or overly sensitive to pain. The pain breakdown goes something like this: 45% complain of painful periods (cramps, back pain, etc.); 37% complain of painful intercourse. At a recent conference on endometriosis, representatives of patient self-help groups from the United Kingdom and North America emphasized how frequently there is a delay in diagnosis. A study revealed that 27% of endometriosis patients complained of symptoms *for six years* before a diagnosis was made. Again, because of the availability of laparoscopy, endometriosis has only been widely diagnosed since the 1970s. The name, as you've probably guessed, comes from the word *endometrium*.

What happens is that endometrial tissue is found outside the uterus in other areas of the body. This tissue develops into small growths, or tumors. (Doctors may also refer to these growths as nodules, lesions, or implants.) These growths are usually benign (meaning noncancerous) and are simply a normal type of tissue in an abnormal location. (There are now some cancers that are being recognized in conjunction with endometriosis, however.)

The most common location of these endometrial growths are in the pelvic region, affecting the ovaries, fallopian tubes, the ligaments supporting the uterus, the perineum, the outer surface of the uterus, and the lining of the pelvic cavity (40–50% of the growths are in the ovaries and fallopian tubes). Sometimes the growths are found in abdominal surgery scars, on the intestines or in the rectum, and on the bladder, vagina, cervix, and vulva. More rare locations include the lung, arm, thigh, and other places outside the abdomen.

Since these growths are in fact pieces of uterine lining, they *behave* like uterine lining, responding to the hormonal cycle and trying to shed every month. These growths, in essence, are blind—they can't see where they are and think they're in the uterus. This is a huge problem during menstruation; when the growths start "shedding," there's no vagina around for them to pass through, so they have nowhere to go. The result is internal bleeding, degeneration of the blood and tissue shed from the growths, inflammation of the surrounding areas, and the formation of scar tissue. Depending on where these growths are located, they can rupture and spread to new areas, cause intestinal bleeding or obstruction (if they're in or near the intestines), or interfere with bladder function (if they're on or near the bladder).

Symptoms

The most common symptoms of endometriosis are pain before and during periods (much worse than normal menstrual cramps), pain during or after intercourse, infertility, and heavy or irregular bleeding. Other symptoms during periods may include fatigue; painful bowel movements; lower back pain; diarrhea and/or constipation; and intestinal upset. If the bladder is involved, there may be painful urination and blood in the urine. Irregular menstrual cycles and heavier flows are also associated with endometriosis, but usually women with severe endometriosis continue to have regular but painful periods.

Some women with endometriosis have no symptoms at all, but infertility affects about 30–40% of endometriosis sufferers and, as the disease progresses, the infertility is often inevitable.

It's important to note that the amount of pain is not necessarily related to the extent or size of the growths. Tiny, or "petechial," growths have been found to be more active in producing prostaglandins, which may explain the significant symptoms that seem to occur with smaller growths. (Prostaglandins are hormonelike chemical substances manufactured by the endometrium. They are thought to be the culprit behind many of the symptoms of endometriosis.)

What causes endometriosis?

Nobody knows the cause of endometriosis. There are a few worthwhile theories, though. One is the theory of *retrograde menstruation*, also known as the *transtubal migration theory*. During menstruation, some of the menstrual tissue backs up through the fallopian tubes, implants in the abdomen and grows. Some researchers believe that *all* women experience some menstrual tissue backup, which is normally eliminated by their immune systems. A malfunctioning immune system or malfunctioning hormones allow this tissue to take root and grow into endometriosis. Another theory suggests that the endometrial tissue is distributed from the uterus to other parts of the body through the lymphatic system or blood system. A genetic theory suggests that it may be carried in the genes of certain families, or that certain families may be predisposed to the disease.

The most interesting theory proposes that remnants of the woman's embryonic tissue (from when she herself was an embryo) may later develop into endometriosis or that some adult tissues retain the ability they had in the embryo *stage* to transform into reproductive tissue under certain circumstances.

The most disturbing theory suggests that endometriosis can be caused by sloppy surgery. Surgical transplantation of endometrial tissue has been cited as the cause in cases where endometriosis is found in abdominal surgery scars. This latter theory is certainly not possible if endometriosis occurs when surgery doesn't!

Diagnosis

The only way to absolutely diagnose endometriosis is through laparoscopy. By moving the laparoscope around, your surgeon can check for any signs of endometrial tissue outside the uterus.

Although many times your doctor can simply feel the endometrial growths in a pelvic exam, no competent physician would confirm the diagnosis without performing a laparoscopy procedure. The bottom line is that if you've been told you have endometriosis, but you *haven't* had a laparoscopy procedure done, go somewhere else for a second opinion, or insist that your doctor perform one. Often, the symptoms of ovarian cancer are identical to endometriosis symptoms. If you've been misdiagnosed with endometriosis due to your doctor's failure to confirm it through laparoscopy, he or she may miss an early diagnosis of ovarian cancer.

A laparoscopy procedure also indicates the locations, extent, and size of the endometrial growths and will help your doctor guide you in treatment decisions and family planning.

Treatment

Treatment for endometriosis has varied over the years but there is still no absolute cure. If you don't have any symptoms and you've decided on adoption, surrogacy, or childfree living, then no treatment is necessary, just regular checkups. If you have only mild symptoms and infertility is *not* a factor, simple painkillers like aspirin or Tylenol may be all that are necessary.

To reverse infertility, *operative laparoscopy* is the best approach. Through a laparoscope, surgery is done with either a laser, cautery, or small surgical instruments. Endometrial implants can be burned off with the laser. (This procedure was shown on The Learning Channel's "The Operation.") However, recurrence is common with this procedure, so you may need to have it repeated if you want future pregnancies. About 40% of women who have an operative laparoscopy procedure will go on to conceive. Even after this more conservative surgery, however, between 20% and 50% of endometriosis patients will need more radical surgery done.

There is a nonsurgical treatment for endometriosis appropriate for women who've decided on childfree living, adoption, or surrogacy. It involves creating a pseudopregnancy with hormonal therapy, used to stop ovulation. This *does* work for as long as you're taking the synthetic hormones, and sometimes the therapy can force endometriosis into remission for months or years. Often, though, when you go off the hormones, the disease comes right back. The hormonal recipe here can include estrogen and progesterone, progesterone alone, *danazol* (a testosterone derivative), and GnRH (gonadotropin-releasing hormone), which creates a psuedomenopause.

For severe symptoms, depending on where the growths are located and their size, your doctor may recommend hysterectomy and removal of the ovaries. This may be an unnecessary procedure and warrants a few separate opinions from other doctors before you agree. Although hysterectomy is is considered a "definitive" cure, research has shown that women who undergo a hysterectomy for endometriosis sometimes experience a recurrence of the disease.

Pregnancy as a Cure

Pregnancy, believe it or not, does cause endometriosis to go into a temporary remission because you don't ovulate when you're pregnant. Furthermore, permanent remission of endometriosis has been known to happen after childbirth; the growths in this case shrink, and the pain associated with the disease stops. The problem is that the longer you have endometriosis, the greater the chance you have of becoming infertile. Furthermore, even under the best of circumstances, women with endometriosis have a higher risk of ectopic pregnancy and miscarriage. One study has found that full-term pregnancies and labor are more difficult when the mother has endometriosis.

Menopause as a cure?

Menopause does generally cure endometriosis (which is why hysterectomy is performed). But a severe case of endometriosis can be reactivated if you begin hormone replacement therapy or continue producing hormones after menopause, which is common. In fact, the oldest woman in whom endometriosis was diagnosed was 78 years old. Some doctors suggest no replacement hormone be given for about 3–9 months after menopause or a hysterectomy procedure.

Fibroids

The medical term for fibroids is *leiomyoma uteri*. Fibroids are benign muscle tumors within the uterus. These are harmless growths that can cause a range of symptoms that include pelvic pain and heavy bleeding during periods. However, just because you have fibroids doesn't mean that you're infertile. Many women with symptomless fibroids experience uncomplicated pregnancies and childbirth. If a fibroid is large enough that it is truly interfering with the implantation of an embryo or the successful duration of a pregnancy, the fibroid can be surgically removed, leaving your reproductive organs intact. Surgical removal of fibroids is called a *myomectomy*. You may need to hunt around for a surgeon that performs these. The best bet is to contact Hysterectomy Educational Resources and Services (HERS) at (215) 667-7757 for the name of a surgeon in your area.

If your fibroids are the culprit behind your infertility and you've decided to adopt or live childfree, you may not need to treat them. Symptomless fibroids can coexist peacefully in your uterus, and since they depend on estrogen to grow, they *will* shrink after menopause (as long as you do not take estrogen therapy). Symptomatic fibroids however, will probably affect your quality of life and will therefore warrant treatment. You could look into hormone therapy, which involves drugs that block estrogen. For severe fibroids, a hysterectomy will be recommended, but often a myomectomy can be done instead, which will preserve your reproductive organs.

Tubal Ligation Reversal

The same surgery that corrects a blocked tube from PID or endometriosis can be used to reverse a tubal ligation in about 60% of the cases. This procedure was demonstrated on The Learning Channel's "The Operation." As long as the *fimbria* within the tube are intact, and there is enough of the tube left for cutting and stitching, the procedure can be a success. The inner canal is sutured, and the outer layer of the tube is reattached. You'll need to have an hysterosalpingogram done about six weeks following the procedure to make sure that the blocked tube is now corrected. Microsurgical techniques in tubal ligation reversals are improving by leaps and bounds. Therefore, the success rates are improving dramatically, too.

Other Structural Abnormalities

Because of the complexity of female anatomy, there's a long list of congenital anatomical defects that can affect a woman's capacity to conceive or sustain a pregnancy. These defects include a double uterus, a double vagina, a separated uterus, an abnormally shaped cervix, uterus, or vagina, and closed or even fused fallopian tubes. All of these defects may not be detected until a fertility workup reveals them through ultrasound or a manual pelvic exam.

Every anatomical oddity is unique and carries options that include reconstructive or repair surgery, or certain kinds of ART procedures that can facilitate biological offspring. You'll need to weigh your options and have a frank discussion with your gynecologist.

Follow-up Care After Surgery

If you've undergone repair surgery for PID, endometriosis, or other structural abnormalities, you will most likely need to have a second hysterosalpingogram done, and possibly a second-look laparoscopy procedure that can check to make sure you're healing properly and that no fresh scarring has occurred.

Most women can expect to feel soreness, have gas, and experience bloating after surgery, but these go away in a few days. You can resume having intercourse once you feel less tender. Pregnancies have been known to occur within the first two cycles after surgery, but many women may continue to experience delays.

Male Factor Infertility

As discussed in chapter 4, close to half of all explained male factor infertility is caused by a structural problem that is *fixable through surgery*. These problems include a varicocele, a varicose vein within the scrotum (contributing to roughly 40% of all male infertility); a blocked tube (accounting for about 3% of all male infertility); and other anatomical defects, such as retrograde ejaculation (about 5%). Infections are occasionally the reason behind poor motility or morphology when a varicocele is ruled out, and are treatable through antibiotics.

When male factor infertility is caused by immunological factors (accounting for about 5% of all male infertility) or hormonal factors (about 2%), treatments are far more tentative and experimental. In these cases, improving sperm quality through various ART techniques may be the only treatment options available. Techniques for improving sperm quality and artificial reproductive technology for males are discussed in chapter 8.

Varicoceles

A varicocele occurs when a varicose vein develops in the spermatic veins leading from the testicles. This happens when the valves in the spermatic veins are damaged, and blood ascending to the heart flows backward instead of engorging the vein. Varicoceles are more common in the left testicle because the veins connect to the renal vein at a right angle, placing more pressure on it.

Infertility is usually the result of a varicocele because the collection of blood surrounding the total area raises the temperature of the testes, which prevents them from producing sperm. Low sperm count, poor motility, and morphology are the results. Diagnosing varicoceles is discussed in chapter 4.

Varicocele repair surgery

This is by far the most common surgical procedure performed to reverse male factor infertility. There are a few different methods available, however, to repair a varicocele.

The least invasive procedure is really an alternative to traditional surgery. It involves the use of an *occlusive*, a device that blocks or plugs up the troublesome vein. In this procedure, an intravenouslike needle is placed through the skin into a large vein in the *neck*, which leads directly to the varicocele, and a springlike coil is dropped down into the vein, which essentially repairs the varicocele. Sometimes a small balloon is used instead of a spring coil, and occasionally a solution is used instead of a coil or balloon, which purposely irritates the varicocele, causing it to scar shut. The procedure is done under a local anesthetic, and you can usually go home a few hours after it's done. You may need to be on a mild painkiller for a few days, and may need to refrain from sexual activity for two to three days following surgery.

Varicoceles can also be repaired under a general anesthetic. Here, you'll go into the hospital as either a day patient or overnight patient, and you'll have the varicocele repaired through an incision in your groin (called a *transinguinal* or *subinguinal* approach). After surgery, you may be uncomfortable for a few days, and you may need to refrain from sexual activity until your incision has healed. Roughly ten days after your surgery, your doctor will want to check your incision to make sure it's healing properly. Then, after about three months, your doctor will request a semen analysis and may want you to deliver a monthly sample until about the twelfth month after your surgery.

About 67% of all men who undergo surgery to repair their varicoceles will see a dramatic improvement in the quality of their semen. Pregnancy rates following surgery are approximately

40% per year, and conception usually occurs withing 6–9 months after the surgery. In short, pregnancy rates triple after a varicocele repair.

Infections and Inflammations

Poor motility or morphology is occasionally caused by infections when a varicocele has been ruled out. When men get infected with STDs such as chlamydia or gonorrhea, if left untreated the infection can either spread deeper inside the reproductive tract or can cause inflammations of the prostate gland (prostatitis), epididydmis (epididymitis) or the testes (orchitis). Other viruses and bacteria that are *not* sexually transmitted can cause inflammation, too.

Prostatitis

Prostatitis literally means "inflammation of the prostate gland due to infection." Most urologists see at least one case of either acute or chronic prostatitis a day. Acute prostatitis means you have a fresh infection and the symptoms come on suddenly. In chronic prostatitis, the condition has existed over a long period of time. Classic symptoms include painful urination, painful ejaculation, and pus and/or blood in the urine. One of the most common causes of prostatitis is coliform bacteria. (*Escherichia coli*, or *e. coli*, is a strain of coliform bacteria.) Coliform bacteria can travel from your colon (where there are always large amounts) into your bladder, urethra, or prostate. When you're constipated, you're especially vulnerable to higher levels of the bacteria, which will hitchhike to your reproductive organs through your lymphatic system or bloodstream.

Another major cause of prostatitis is STDs. Chlamydia, gonorrhea, trichomonas vaginalis ("trich"), and even vaginal yeast infections (which are technically not STDs but can be passed on to the male) can cause this infection. Bacteria such as staphylococcus (causing common colds and a garden variety of ailments) accounts for roughly 5% of all prostatitis.

Prostatitis will affect your fertility for as long as you're infected, causing poor motility and poor morphology. Treatment is simple: antibiotics. Your doctor will first need to culture your infection by either taking some prostatic fluid (done during a rectal exam, where the doctor puts pressure on the gland, and causes the fluid to come out of your urethra), or in some cases, a culture can be obtained from a urine and a semen sample. Once the right bacterium is identified, you'll be placed on antibiotics for about 3–6 weeks and will then need to repeat your semen analysis and urinalysis to make sure the infection has cleared. Your partner must also be treated to make sure that you aren't passing bacteria back and forth.

Epididymitis

When the epididymis becomes inflamed, it causes swelling, pain, burning urination, and even discharge from the urethra. Blockage of the ejaculatory ducts can result, causing either low or no sperm counts. The most common causes of epididymitis are chlamydia and gonorrhea. If caught early enough, antibiotics will cure the infection without leaving any damage. However, if the infection is left untreated, it could cause permanent scarring and blockages in the epididymal ducts.

Repairing the blockage is only possible through microsurgical resection of the epididymis under a general anesthetic. This procedure is called an *epididymovasostomy*. The blocked section is cut out and the ejaculatory duct is reconnected. The best way to explain the surgery is to compare it to reattaching a long rope or chord that was once severed. This is an open surgical procedure done on the scrotum. (See Figure 7 for a diagram of what the procedure involves.) Repairing blockages in the ejaculatory ducts can be done with a transurethral procedure, however. There is some risk: If the valve leading to the bladder is harmed in any way, surgery could result in retrograde ejaculation or even incontinence.

Rarely, infection can cause blockages in the vas deferens. A *vasovasostomy*, similar to an epididymovasostomy, can repair the obstruction. But usually obstruction of the vas deferens is *deliberate*, caused by a vasectomy. To reverse a vasectomy, a vasovasostomy is considered highly effective, with pregnancy rates as high as 70% after the reversal. The best candidates for vasectomy reversals are those who had their vasectomy within the last ten years. (The Learning Channel's "The Operation" showed this procedure.)

Orchitis

Orchitis, inflammation of the testes, can be dangerous to an adult male's fertility because it can

Diagram of the Epididymovasostomy procedure

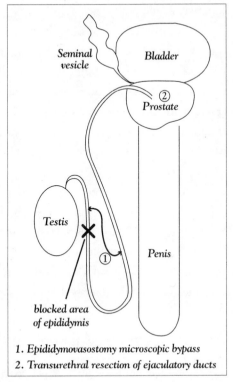

1. *Epididymovasostomy microscopic bypass*
2. *Transurethral resection of ejaculatory ducts*

Figure 9.
Source: Keith Jarvi, M.D., F.R.C.S.(C), 1994.

cause permanent, irreversible sterility. When orchitis occurs prior to puberty, a man's testicular function should not be affected.

Viral infections are usually the cause of orchitis, the most notorious of which are the mumps. Roughly 25% of men with mumps get pain and swelling in one or both testicles. In this case, not only is the swelling of the testes dangerous, but the mumps virus also directly attacks the testes and can destroy their ability to make sperm. The amount of swelling, however, does not have bearing on the amount of sperm damage that occurs. In fact, some men can fully recover from the mumps and go on to father children, while others remain infertile. Testicular failure is easily diagnosed through a blood test, which will show high levels of FSH and LH, signs that the testes are failing.

The mumps are certainly not the only disease that causes orchitis. Syphilis, tuberculosis, pancreatitis, hepatitis, mononucleosis, and smallpox can cause orchitis as well. However, you can have any of the above diseases, including the mumps, and not suffer from orchitis.

Symptoms of orchitis include a discharge of pus or mucus from the penis, dull twinges of pain in the testicles, and lower back pain. Early diagnosis and prompt treatment of orchitis prevent further testicular damage.

Treating Common Anatomical Problems

There are some common anatomical problems that are either congenital or can result from other diseases or injury. If treatment isn't available, solutions to infertility are!

Retrograde ejaculation

As discussed in chapter 4, this is a condition where the bladder neck doesn't completely close during ejaculation, causing the semen to be propelled backward into the bladder. Men with diabetes or a history of testicular cancer can be prone to this.

There is no treatment for retrograde ejaculation, but there is a solution to infertility. Men with this problem can still father a child by having their sperm retrieved from their urine and then inseminated into their partner. The female cycle is monitored closely so insemination can take place during ovulation. Roughly two days before "retrieval day," a man must refrain from ejaculation. The day of retrieval, he must take two sodium bicarbonate tablets with water every two hours, eight hours prior to retrieval. The sodium creates a more alkaline environment in the bladder, which allows the sperm to survive longer.

Thirty minutes before retrieval, the man empties his bladder completely. Then he ejaculates either through masturbation or regular intercourse (intercourse may not be possible if he lives far from his doctor's office). He then delivers a urine sample to his doctor's office or lab, where the sperm is washed (see chapter 4), separated from the the urine (by being put into a solution), and inseminated into his partner. The average couple goes through about six of these insemination procedures and, amazingly, six out of seven will conceive.

Undescended testicles

A small percentage of all male babies are born with one or both testes still inside the abdomen. This is known as *cryptorchidism*. Out of all the babies born with cryptorchidism, the majority of the testes descend by themselves within about four months. Less than 1 percent of babies whose cryptorchidism persists may be treated with a surgical procedure known as *orchipexy*. The surgery usually is not performed until six months after birth to allow for a natural reversal of the condition. Here, the testes are manually delivered out of the abdomen during surgery (usually a laparotomy procedure) so that they will lie normally in the scrotum.

The reason why this condition can lead to sterility is because sperm cannot be produced within the warm temperatures of the abdomen. If this condition remains untreated, a male is at high risk of developing testicular cancer. Sometimes, even after treatment a male still may have very low sperm counts. In this case, intrauterine insemination (IUI) may be an option. Up to 10% of men with no sperm have missing ducts. An uncommon clinical condition, affecting the lungs and pancreas, is a disease called cystic fibrosis (CF). The gene for CF is the most common cause of missing duct. If you have missing ducts, it's crucial that you be tested for CF.

Blocked or missing ducts

Men born to women who took DES (see chapter 1) can be prone to a variety of congenital defects that include a missing or defective vas deferens or missing seminal vesicles. In these cases, the semen volume is low and may be accompanied by low or no sperm counts.

To date, there is no way to replace missing ducts, but a procedure known as *sperm aspiration* (for men who have blocked or absent vas deferens or who have had vasectomies) can allow a man to father a child. Here, immature sperm are surgically removed from the epididydmis (through an incision in the scrotum) and cultured in a laboratory, then used in an IVF procedure with the female partner's egg. (See chapter 8 for details on IVF.) Other than this option, men with these problems must seek out other parenting options, such as adoption or donor insemination, or choose a childfree lifestyle.

Hypospadias and epispadias

A common congenital problem involves an abnormal urethral opening. Here the opening of the urethra on the penis is somewhere other than at the tip: the underside (known as *hypospadias*) or upperside (known as *epispadias*). Sperm production is fine, but when ejaculated it won't be deposited directly into the cervix. This is easily corrected through plastic surgery, where a new opening at the the tip of the penis is constructed and the old opening is closed up.

Torsion

One of the reasons why the testes are ultrasensitive to pain is to protect them from serious injury. Injury to even one testicle can cause torsion, when the testicle twists inside the scrotum. Pelvic surgeries such as hernia repair or bladder surgery can also cause testicular torsion. Torsion can be surgically repaired if it's caught early enough, but if left untreated the testicle (or both testes) shrinks and withers away (atrophy) to the point where it is the size of a pea. When atrophy occurs, there is no treatment and men with this problem will need to seek other parenting options.

Treating Immunological Infertility

As discussed in chapter 4, some male-factor infertility is caused by antisperm antibodies; the sperm is coated with antibodies that harm the sperm, causing poor motility or failure for the sperm to recognize or penetrate the egg.

Women can also form antibodies to a partner's sperm, causing the sperm to clump together around the cervix or to have poor motility. Generally, though, infection or inflammation is the main trigger of male-produced antisperm antibodies, while a vasectomy procedure is also cited as a major cause. Sperm ingestion can lead to immunological infertility as well, which is discussed in chapter 2.

If there are only a few antisperm antibodies in your system, this shouldn't create a barrier to fertility. However, if the antibodies are present in large numbers, you've got a big problem.

Treatment

To date, treatment for immunological infertility is not very successful. Here, corticosteriods (anti-inflammatory drugs such as methylprednisolone, prednisone, or dexamethasone) are used to suppress the immune system. The theory is that when the immune system is suppressed, the antisperm antibodies will be less lethal on the sperm.

Unfortunately, there are some very unpleasant side-effects to these drugs, which include rashes, irritability, depression, indigestion, weight gain, and fluid retention. Pregnancy rates on these drugs hover around 30%; however, the best way to reverse infertility is to combine the drug therapy with either IUI or IVF, both discussed in chapter 8 .

Premature Testicular Failure

Men who receive chemotherapy or radiation therapy to the testes, or who are exposed to known environmental toxins in the workplace, are at high risk of suffering from testicular failure. This is when your testicles shut down and stop producing sperm. Common cancers in younger men include Hodgkin's disease, non-Hodgkin's lymphoma, leukemia, testicular cancer, and melanoma. Prior to your treatment, you should bank significant quantities of your own sperm (waiting 2–4 days between samples) if you do not yet have a family. Your sperm can be frozen indefinitely until you're ready for it to be inseminated into your partner.

A Word About Sexual Dysfunction

A significant portion of male factor infertility is caused by sexual disorders rather than physiological problems. Therapy is available for a variety of problems that include premature ejaculation, anejaculation, impotence, and poor libido. Ask your urologist or family doctor to recommend you to a sex therapist or counselor if a physical cause for your dysfunction is ruled out. In many cases, sexual dysfunction is rooted in emotional trauma that can be treated through psychiatric therapy. Inappropriate emotional or physical stimulation can also result in sexual dysfunction.

Because of the way humans are built, while many women are also sexually dysfunctional (not able to climax and so on), female sexual performance does not correspond to reduced fertility the same way that male sexual performance does.

Secondary Infertility

It is possible to be infertile after having one or more biological children. This is known as *secondary infertility*. *Primary infertility* refers to couples who have never conceived. Secondary infertility carries unique frustrations because couples can't help saying, "We've reproduced once, why can't we reproduce again?" Couples experiencing secondary infertility will go through the same workups discussed in chapters 4 and 5. There are some common causes of secondary infertility that you may want to rule out first, though, before proceeding with a battery of tests.

- *Varicoceles*. As men get into their late 30s and early 40s, varicoceles can develop. Get this checked out early.
- *Prostate health*. In addition to prostatitis, overall prostate health tends to deteriorate as men age. Make sure you don't neglect this aspect of your yearly physical exam.
- *Endometriosis*. This is cited as the most frequent cause of secondary infertility in women.
- *PID*. This can worsen with time if the original bacteria causing PID was never treated.

Other Factors to Consider

Age
Even five years can make a big difference in a woman's fertility cycle and a man's sperm count. Many couples have one child and then space out the next one to coincide with their first child's school schedule. For busy career couples, this spacing helps make two children more manageable.

If you've started your family later in life (after 35) and are considering more children, you might look into banking your sperm and freezing previously retrieved eggs to be used in an ART procedure just in case you run into problems.

Scarring after childbirth
If you had a difficult first labor and childbirth experience and suffered from a bacterial infection after childbirth, scarring may be the culprit behind your infertility now. A laparoscopy would confirm whether this is the problem.

Stress
Stress increases enormously after one child, which can affect ovulation and sperm production. See chapter 2 for more information.

Strenuous exercise and weight loss
Many women will overdo it in the gym in a mad scramble to reclaim their slim figures after childbirth. This can affect ovulation for future pregnancies.

Whether your fertility problem is female factor or male factor in origin, if treatment of your health problem hasn't resulted in pregnancy (including the use of fertility drugs to *induce* ovulation), fertility drugs may be used to *enhance* ovulation in cases where ART procedures are being used. The next chapter is all about the uses and the risks of these drugs.

If fertility drugs are not an option, you may need to consider other options, such as surrogacy, adoption, or childfree living. Surrogacy is discussed in chapter 8; options to biological parenting are discussed in chapter 10.

7

All About Fertility Drugs

As we've seen in chapters 4, 5, and 6, fertility drugs may be prescribed to *many* women and to *some* men for a variety of hormonal problems and unexplained infertility. Even women who ovulate regularly may start using fertility drugs if they're undergoing any sort of assisted reproductive technology (ART) procedure, such as in vitro fertilization (IVF) or gamete intrafallopian transfer (GIFT).

In the majority of cases, fertility drugs are used to induce ovulation in anovulatory women (see chapters 3 and 5) or to increase follicle stimulation in women undergoing ART (see chapter 8) procedures. Only a tiny segment of fertility drug users are male (see chapter 4). Therefore, this chapter is directed primarily at the female reader; the last section of the chapter discusses the use of fertility drugs in men.

Some women's organizations would argue that fertility drugs would not be as widely used if the majority of patients using the drugs *were* male. They compare the widespread DES (diethylstilbestrol) and other disastrous women's health products such as the Dalkon Shield or thalidomide (not available in the United States). All of these products were introduced onto the market without adequately researching the long-term consequences. A large portion of this chapter focuses on the known risks of fertility drugs and explores some of the unknown potential risks.

Fertility Drugspeak

It's a little difficult to make an informed decision about fertility drugs unless you understand what you're really taking. Unfortunately, many specialists will give you a prescription with only a brief explanation of side effects and when to take your medication. Worse, even if your doctor explains what the drugs are, distinguishing between the generic drug names and brand names of all these products can be pretty overwhelming. Here's an explanation in plain English.

For most women, ovulation induction will involve the drug *clomiphene citrate* (CC). Popular brand names of CC are Clomid and Serophene. CC is an *analogue*, which, in the language of pharmacology, means "chemical imposter." To the body, CC looks like it belongs, which enables it to sneak in to your system and *block* estrogen in the body. This is also referred to as an anti-estrogen. High levels of estrogen prevent ovulation from occurring, and when the estrogen is blocked out *completely*, your ovaries respond by making more follicles than they normally would, in an effort to make the estrogen it thinks is missing. (Follicles secrete estrogen, as explained in chapter 3.) CC is discussed in detail further below.

Some women will be offered more potent drugs, known as *gonadotropins*, which are administered by injection. Gonadotropins are sex hormones secreted by the pituitary gland; FSH Follicle stimulating hormone (FSH), luteinizing hormone (LH) or human chorionic gonadotropin (HCG) are all gonadotropins. To date, FSH and LH can only be extracted from one source: the urine of menopausal women. In menopause, FSH and LH levels are naturally high to compensate for retiring ovaries. When FSH and LH are extracted from the urine and refined, they make up a product called *human menopausal gonadotropin* (HMG).

There are different *variants* of HMG. The most popular form of HMG is a *menotropin*, which contains equal parts of FSH and LH. The most popular brand name menotropin is Pergonal. (In Canada and the United Kingdom, another brand of menotropin is Humegon.) Some drug companies make *urofollitropin*, a strain of HMG that consists of mostly FSH, with very little LH in it at all. Metrodin is the most popular brand-name urofollitropin.

For the majority of women offered HMG, they'll take the menotropin (Pergonal or Humegon), which contains both FSH and LH. For women with polycystic ovarian syndrome, they'll most likely be offered the urofollitropin (after a failed attempt on CC), since they'll already have high levels of LH in their systems.

When you're on HMG (whether it's menotropin or urofollitropin) you'll also receive injections of HCG. HCG is a hormone secreted by the developing placenta during a pregnancy. (HCG secretion is what a home pregnancy test looks for in your urine.) When you're not yet pregnant, however, HCG will cause your developing follicle (at this point known as the corpus luteum) to secrete enough estrogen and progesterone to maintain a pregnancy.

Your doctor may want to put you on a *gonadotropin-releasing hormone* (GnRH) *analogue* prior to starting you on CC or HMG. Popular brand names of these drugs are Lupron, Synarel (which is in a nasal spray format), Suprefact, and Zolidex. These drugs block your *entire* natural cycle by blocking out GnRH, secreted by your hypothalamus gland to kick-start the pituitary gland into secreting FSH and LH. By giving the analogue, the drug removes the control of GnRH from your hypothalamus and takes over that function instead. GnRH analogues are rather complicated drugs. Some doctors feel that controlling the cycle completely through artificial means is more effective than mixing artificial hormones with natural hormones.

Finally, there are some very specific hormonal disorders that can interfere with a normal ovulation cycle, such as hyperprolactinemia (see chapter 5) or a GnRH deficiency. In these cases, you'll be offered an exact replacement of the hormone you're not producing. These drugs, such as bromocriptine or Lutrepulse, are also discussed further on.

Who Needs Treatment?

People who are offered fertility drugs fall into four groups:
- Women who are anovulatory. This includes all of the hormonal disorders discussed in chapter 5, as well as women with polycystic ovarian syndrome (PCO) (see chapters 5 and 6).
- Women who have complete ovulatory failure, a condition known as *hypogonadotrophic hypogonadism*. Surgery or radiotherapy for a pituitary tumor can cause this condition.
- Women who are in an ART program such as IVF or GIFT. In this case, while you may be ovulating regularly, in order for IVF or GIFT to succeed, you need to have *several* mature follicles in each cycle. This gives your doctor better "pickings" for the petri dishes. Your ovaries will be stimulated with fertility drugs for these procedures.
- Couples with unexplained infertility.
- Men who have certain hormonal disorders that respond to fertility drugs. See the section on "Drugs Used in Male Fertility Therapy" later in this chapter.

Operation Ovulation Induction

If you're not ovulating regularly, at least one or more of the drugs discussed in this section will be offered to you in the hope that your ovulation will be restored long *enough* for you to conceive. None of the medications described in this chapter is intended to be used as a long-term therapy, however. The dosages, side effects, and risks of each of these drugs are thoroughly covered in the following section. I also discuss the diagnostic tests you'll need prior to beginning treatment, as well as the tests you'll need while you're on the drugs. Finally, I identify those women who should not be taking these medications. If you're taking the drugs as part of an ART program, please refer to the section "Operation Egg Retrieval" later in this chapter. In general, your treatment will differ only at ovulation, where your eggs will be retrieved and then either put back inside you, or inside a host uterus (done in the case of oocyte donation, discussed in chapter 8.)

Clomiphene Citrate (CC)

Clomiphene citrate (CC) is the most common drug used for ovulation induction. Clomid and Serophene are its most popular brand names. CC comes in the form of an oral tablet and is taken for five days starting from the fifth day of your period (whether it's natural or induced). When you stop the drug, you'll get your LH surge, which stimulates ovulation and provides you with a high-quality luteal phase. Using a 28-day cycle as an example, you'd start on 50 milligrams of CC on day 5 of your cycle. You'd take it until about day 9 and then go off it. This will induce ovulation about 6–0 days later (or roughly day 15–19 of the cycle). You'll need to keep track of your basal body temperature throughout this process and will probably have your serum progesterone levels taken around this time to monitor whether the drug is working. If you don't menstruate at all, you'll first have your period induced by a progesterone supplement before starting CC. If 50 milligrams doesn't do the trick, the dosage will be gradually increased to roughly 100 milligrams. (Women have been known to go as high as 250 milligrams per day for five or more days per cycle, but this really isn't advised.)

It's absolutely crucial that your doctor puts you on 50 milligrams, the *lowest possible dosage*. If ovulation isn't taking place, your dosage will increase to 100 milligrams. If ovulation still isn't oc-curring, you should be taken off CC. Going to a higher dosage is not recommeded because there may be adverse reactions, Instead, you may be offered HMG, a more powerful drug.

It can take a few months to establish the right dose, but once you're on an effective dose (be it 50, 75, or 100 milligrams), you'll be on CC for roughly six months. If the drug doesn't work in six months, it most likely *won't*. You see, the likelihood of conception *diminishes* with each CC cycle you do. The six-month cycle takes into account the fact that you need a couple of cycles to establish the right dosage. Once that happens, three cycles of CC is about the maximum most doctors will allow.

CC can also cause your cervical mucus to thicken, which can create another fertility barrier. As discussed in chapters 3, 4, and 5, high-quality cervical mucus is necessary in order for the sperm to reach the egg. To make sure the sperm are surviving in the cervix, a postcoital test (see chapter 5) should be done after you begin CC.

It's important that the cause for your anovulatory disorder is found first, and that you've completed both a male and female workup (see chapters 4 and 5). In other words, you must not take the drug unless you and your partner have been seen by a fertility specialist. Helping yourself to your sister's supply of CC, for example, is a *really* bad idea!

CC works well for women who ovulate *occasionally* rather than never. It is useless in improving ovulation for women who ovulate regularly, or in inducing ovulation in women who have primary ovarian failure, which would be indicated by high levels of FSH in your blood—the result of premature or natural menopause, for example.

Costs

Clomiphene is the cheapest of the fertility drugs, costing about $25 per cycle as of 1995. Some insurance plans may cover the costs of these drugs, while others may consider these drugs "experimental." You can try to get your doctor to write a letter, which in some cases facilitates more coverage. In other cases, some drug companies have limited funds that they make available to patients to help them pay for one or two cycles' worth of CC. In general, most CC patients (even Canadians) should not count on getting these funds.

A *word about storage*

You'll need to store your drugs in a dark, dry place. Light or moisture may affect their potency. If the drugs are not working in the first two cycles, explore the possibility that storage, rather than dosage, may be the problem. For example, bathrooms are typically the worst place to store them, yet most people will choose this area.

What are the odds?

About 60% of all women on CC ovulate, while about 30% do get pregnant within the first three months of treatment. There is also about a 10% chance of conceiving twins if you take the drug and, in fact, the risk of miscarriage *drops* (because the drug also improves the luteal phase, there is a greater chance that the pregnancy "sticks").

Who's not a clomiphene citrate candidate?

You cannot take clomiphene citrate if you have any of the following conditions:

- Suspected pregnancy. To avoid taking clomiphene during a pregnancy, make sure you keep a basal body temperature chart or another chart (see chapter 3) so you can keep track of your cycles. Then, you should not restart clomiphene citrate if your period is late and rule out or confirm the pregnancy before you start your next clomiphene cycle.

- Uncontrolled thyroid disorder or adrenal disorder. If you've been successfully treated for one of these conditions, then it's fine to take CC.
- Pituitary tumor or another organic intracranial lesion.
- Liver disease or a history of liver disease. Women with liver problems won't absorb and break down the drug properly, nor should they risk pregnancy without discussing the risks with an internist.)
- Abnormal uterine bleeding that hasn't yet been investigated or has no known cause. This suggests that you have too much estrogen in your system already, so the last thing you need is MORE!
- Ovarian cysts or enlargement of one or both ovaries that is NOT due to polycystic ovarian syndrome. Because the drug causes more follicles to ripen, there's a higher risk of developing ovarian cysts or enlarged ovaries. This is discussed more below.
- Depression or a history of depression. These drugs can cause symptoms of depression that can aggravate a preexisting history.
- Fibroids. The increase in estrogen can stimulate the fibroids to grow, which is not dangerous to your general health but could interefere with a pregnancy. Discuss the risks with your doctor further so you can make an informed decision.

You should not take clomiphene citrate unless:
- Your partner has a clean bill of health from his workup (see chapter 4).
- You have been charting your cycles and have a clear understanding of how your own menstrual cycle works (see chapter 3).
- You have had a full workup yourself, including a full physical, pelvic exam, negative Pap smear, blood tests that check your estrogen and progesterone levels at key phases in the cycle, a clean hysterosalpingogram (meaning your tubes are open), and an endometrial biopsy that determines whether or not you have a luteal phase deficiency. (All these are discussed in chapter 5.)

If you're over 40 . . .
As you age, your risk of endometrial cancer (which is an estrogen-dependent cancer) goes up, so high levels of estrogen can put you at further risk. Discuss your risk profile with your doctor *before*

you go on clomiphene citrate. (For example, are you overweight? Do you have a family history of this cancer?) You may need to have a dilatation and curettage (D & C) done before you start your clomiphene citrate, but in many cases, an endometrial biopsy is enough. A D & C will rule out any early warning signs of endometrial cancer. Finally, you should have a mammogram done prior to starting clomiphene citrate, and/or prior to trying to conceive.

Side effects

You may recognize many of the clomiphene citrate side-effects from your days on oral contraceptives. Most of these side effects have to do with increased levels of estrogen in your system. You may even confuse the side effects of clomiphene with premenstrual symptoms or even pregnancy symptoms. The most serious side effect is ovarian enlargement. This occurs in approximately 1 in 7 women on CC. Careful monitoring through ultrasound will help to isolate this symptom before it becomes dangerous. (Severe ovarian enlargement that comes on suddenly rather than gradually is called *hyperstimulation syndrome* and is discussed separately below.) Hot flashes resembling menopausal symptoms occur in roughly 1 in 10 women, while roughly 1 in 15 women will experience diarrhea, constipation, or bloating.

About 1 in 50 women on CC will experience stomach upset, breast tenderness, nausea and vomiting, nervousness, insomnia, and vision problems, while about 1 in 100 will experience headaches, dizziness and light-headedness, increased urination, depression, fatigue, skin changes, abnormal uterine bleeding, weight gain, ovarian cysts, and reversible hair loss. Some of these women may also experience cramping during ovulation (known as *mittelschmerz*). *Warning: The higher the dose, the greater the risk of ovarian enlargement and vision problems.*

It should also be noted that CC can interfere with the production of high-quality mid-cycle cervical mucus, creating another barrier to fertility while solving another.

A word about visual problems

In about 1 in 50 women on CC, visual problems may develop shortly after beginning treatment. The symptoms usually involve blurring or seeing spots or flashes (scintillating scotomata), and the problem seems to be directly linked to dosage; the greater your dosage, the worse your vision symptoms may be. On the more severe side, vision symptoms can include double vision (diplopia), seeing rings of light (phosphenes), oversensitivity to light (photophobia), decreased visual acuity, loss of peripheral vision, and spatial distortion. If you experience these symptoms, discontinue CC immediately. Your vision should return to normal within a few days. Often symptoms will first appear or will be exacerbated by a brightly lit environment. Ophthalmologists have reported noticeable changes in the eyes of patients on CC. *In other words, these vision symptoms are real and not imagined.*

If you operate machinery, work under conditions where the lighting is poor, or are doing any significant amounts of driving, be on alert for these symptoms. If you must discontinue CC because of these symptoms, you must follow up with a visit to an ophthalmologist.

A word about periods

While you're on CC, your periods may become lighter or heavier than usual. There may also be a 2–3 day delay in your period, which may make you suspect pregnancy. You may also have heavier cramping.

Don't confuse side effects with pregnancy symptoms

Obviously, many of the CC side effects mimic some of the symptoms of pregnancy: nausea and vomiting, delayed period, breast tenderness, dizziness, and so on. Whenever you experience any of these symptoms or side effects, report them to your doctor and have a pregnancy test done.

Risks

To date, no increase in birth defects has been reported with CC; your risk is comparable to that of the general population. However, there is the risk of a *multiple pregnancy*, which carries greater risks, such as premature delivery and increased complications. In unassisted conceptions, the risk of a multiple pregnancy is about 1 in 80; with pregnancies conceived on CC, the risk is about 1 in 20, a *significant* increase! Out of all the pregnancies reported on CC, 90% were single fetuses and 10% were twins. Less than 1% were triplets or more. See the separate section on multiple pregnancies for more details.

CC carries some more severe risks, which include an ovarian disorder known as *hyperstimulation syndrome*. This is discussed in a separate section below, since HMG carries the same risks.

Finally, there have also been ectopic pregnancies reported in CC pregnancies, but this risk is not any greater than in the general, fertile population. Technically though, some literature lists ectopic pregnancy as a "risk" because because CC cannot *prevent* an ectopic pregnancy from occurring.

If you need to discontinue treatment...

You may be able to resume treatment with CC after taking a break from it for three months or so. Discuss this possibility with your doctor. Reestablishing treatment with CC depends on the severity of your side effects, your overall health, and the dosage. Keep in mind, though, that long-term use of CC is *NOT* recommended.

A *word about monitoring*

Since the point of CC is to induce ovulation just long enough for a conception to occur, it's crucial that you keep track of your basal body temperature throughout the cycle. Once you start CC, your doctor should take your FSH levels around day 2 or 3 of the cycle via a blood test, and retake your FSH levels around days 10-12 to see if the levels have doubled. If they have, then all is going well, and you may continue your CC cycle. On day 10 or 11 of the cycle, a transvaginal ultrasound (see chapter 5) should also be done to monitor the maturation of your follicles. This monitoring is essential in order to keep watch for any adverse enlargement of your ovaries. Monitoring the cycle will also help you time your intercourse more exactly so you can conceive.

If your doctor gives you a CC prescription and tells you not to come back for a month, *go elsewhere. This is a sign that he or she doesn't understand how to administer the drug.* CC, again, must be given only to women whose partners had a full workup, and who themselves have been screened for other possible causes of female fertility, such as blocked or scarred fallopian tubes. See the separate section on monitoring below for more details.

Human Menopausal Gonadotropin (HMG)

As discussed in the DrugSpeak section HMG comes under the generic drug names *urofollitropin* (Metrodin), which is pure FSH and is reserved for PCO women or *menotropin* (Pergonal or Humegon), which is pure FSH and LH in equal parts. Women will only require HMG treatment to induce ovulation if they're *not* responding to clomiphene citrate. Women who are more likely to be offered HMG are those who have very low estrogen levels to begin with, those who have PCO (these women will get urofollitropin), and those who are undergoing an ART procedure (see the section "Operation Egg Retrieval"). If you're offered HMG without first being put on clomiphene citrate, *question it!* This is *not* a standard or recommended approach. The general scenario is to do about three cycles of CC and then graduate to HMG if you're not responding.

A *pain in the butt*

HMG can be administered only via an intramuscular injection, usually in the buttocks or thighs. Because HMG is a protein, if it's taken orally it would be digested in the stomach and would not be effectively absorbed into your body. In addition, the drug needs to be individualized for each woman to accommodate her from cycle to cycle. These injections can be self-administered or administered by your partner at home (your doctor will show him how to do it). Otherwise, you'll need to make daily trips to the doctor's office.

How a typical HMG cycle works

A few days after your period or day 2 or 3 of your cycle, you'll go for your first baseline ultrasound, and then have your estradiol, FSH, and LH levels checked. Then, if all is well, you'll go for your first HMG injection. (All women will have these injections daily.) Assuming a 28-day cycle, you'll begin to take two ampules of HMG until day 5 or 6. At that point, you'll return to your doctor's office for an ultrasound and a check of your estradiol levels. Your doctor will then carefully monitor your cycle by taking daily blood samples to check hormone levels, and doing daily transvaginal ultrasounds to determine the quality, quantity and maturity of your follicles. If too many follicles develop, the doctor will stop the treatment until the next cycle to avoid a grossly multiple birth. Basically, the HMG dosage is adjusted to the number of follicles developing, your estrogen levels, and so on. When the ultrasound reveals mature eggs of 1.8 centimeters, you'll be injected with *human chorionic gonadotropin* (HCG), which stimulates LH, creating your LH surge. Ovulation should occur 24–36 hours later. From a pharmacological standpoint, HCG is actually the same thing as "pituitary LH," and it's given to you because it keeps your corpus luteum working longer secreting progesterone and estrogen. (Profasi and A.P.L. are brand names of HCG, but there are others.) A typical cycle involves anywhere from 7–12 HMG injections.

Who isn't an HMG candidate?

For the most part, if you can't take clomiphene citrate, then you *definitely* can't take HMG. The only exceptions are women with liver disorders. Because HMG is *not* digested but injected, your liver doesn't need to break down the drug, so there's no reason you can't take HMG. You also cannot be on HMG if you have primary or premature ovarian failure or have had bad reactions to HMG or clomiphene citrate in the past. If you have a history of pulmonary or vascular disorders, you should be aware that HMG can can cause both pulmonary and vascular complications, but you are not considered at higher risk for these symptoms than are those in the general population. If you're over 40, the drug can increase the risk of endometrial cancer. You should rule out endometrial cancer risks before you begin HMG.

Finally, you shouldn't be on HMG unless you and your partner have already been screened for other fertility problems, you've had a diagnostic laparoscopy, and you've already had an unsuccessful bout with CC. HMG should be the last resort for ovulation induction.

Side effects

The most serious side effects of HMG are enlarged ovaries, which can range from moderate to severe. When severe ovarian enlargement comes on suddenly, this is known as hyperstimulation syndrome, a side effect of clomiphene citrate. *Enlarged ovaries occur in about 20% of all women on HMG, accompanied by abdominal distension and pain.* You should stop treatment immediately. Other side effects are abdominal pain; rash or swelling at the injection site; headache; gastrointestinal complaints; fever or flulike symptoms (fever, chills, nausea, and vomiting); breast tenderness and skin reactions; rapid heart rate (tachycardia); and rapid breathing.

As mentioned above, pulmonary disorders such as lung collapse or acute respiratory distress syndrome, in which the fluid builds up into the lung tissue, can occur. Bleeding in the abdominal region (hemoperitoneum) can also develop because HMG causes your blood vessel walls to become porous.

Periods may also be heavier, with heavier cramping, and you may feel cramping during ovulation. If your periods are delayed, you must rule out a pregnancy before you continue. As with CC, some of these side effects can be confused with pregnancy symptoms; don't conclude you are pregnant until you check it out.

Side effects of HCG

When you stop your HMG injections and begin your HCG injections, you may experience headache, irritability, restlessness, fatigue, depression, or a swelling or rash at the injection site. Some women may continue to experience side effects from HMG, too, but the above list refers exclusively to side effects of HCG. If you've demonstrated a past allergy or adverse reaction to HCG, you shouldn't be on the drug a second time.

HMG storage

If you're self-injecting at home (your doctor will show you how), the drug should be stored in the refrigerator. HMG comes in a freeze-dried form, with a separate liquid that's added just before injection. Once you mix the two substances together, you must take the drug *immediately*. You can't mix them up an hour before you plan to take it, and you can't put the leftover drug in the refrigerator to take the next day.

The costs

This is an expensive drug, costing well over $1,000 per cycle as of 1995. Fewer drug plans cover HMG than clomiphene citrate. You may be able to obtain coverage if your doctor writes a letter to your drug plan or insurer. As with clomiphene, some drug companies make limited funding available to patients to help cover the costs of one or two cycles. But for the majority of patients on HMG, you're on your own. Again because of the expense, inconvenience and side effects of this drug, HMG should be used as a last resort.

The odds

In the end, while 75% women will ovulate with HMG, the pregnancy rate on the drug drastically varies: 20–80% of all HMG cycles will end in pregnancy. Twins occur in 20–40% of all pregnancies that result from HMG.

The Risks

The risks of HMG are similar those of CC: multiple pregnancies (occurring in 20–40% of all HMG pregnancies), ovarian hyperstimulation syndrome (discussed separately below), and an increased risk of ovarian cancer. Ectopic pregnancies have been reported but, again, this risk is not any greater than it is to the general, fertile population.

GnRH Analogues

Some doctors will want put you on a *GnRH analogue*—a GnRH "copycat" that takes over GnRH production for your hypothalamus, blocking its communication link to the pituitary gland. The result is that your entire hormonal axis is shut down. The shutdown occurs because your hypothalamus thinks: "Oh, I don't need to release GnRH; it's already here." The pituitary gland therefore has its "hands tied"; it cannot release FSH or LH until it receives GnRH. Your body goes into a kind of postmenopausal or prepubertal state, enabling your doctor to control your entire cycle with drugs. Some brand names of GnRH analogues are Lupron, Synarel (in a nasal spray form), Suprefact, and Zolidex.

To date, these drugs are not intended by the FDA as fertility drugs per se, but they are used nonetheless by many specialists. Some believe that a controlled cycle allows HMG to work more effectively.

These drugs are often used to treat other problems, including fibroids and endometriosis. The analogues are administered by a pump that acts like a normal hypothalamus. The pump is discussed later in this chapter, since it is also used to treat women with a GnRH deficiency. In this case, pure GnRH, rather than an analogue, is prescribed.

Ovarian Hyperstimulation Syndrome (OHSS)

This is a condition that develops when the ovaries are overstimulated by either CC or HMG, and therefore enlarge suddenly and overproduce follicles. The condition is rarely seen with CC and is more common with HMG. The symptoms of OHSS are abdominal bloating or distension, discomfort, nausea (which may be mistaken for morning sickness), and sometimes difficulty breathing (which can be confused with dyspnea).

This condition is thankfully quite rare when the dose is low and the drug is used correctly, but the higher the dose and the longer you're on the drug, the higher the risk of OHSS. Women with PCO are more prone to OHSS than other women on the drugs. In general, roughly 6% of all PCO women on urofollitropin will develop OHSS, but only about 1.3% of women on menotropin will develop the condition.

If this condition is left undetected, hospitalization may be necessary. Keep in mind that virtually no specialist will put you on fertility drugs without monitoring your cycle via ultrasounds and blood samples throughout. One of the key reasons why monitoring is done is to prevent this condition from developing.

Monitoring an Induced Cycle

Whether you're taking CC or HMG, you must be monitored (on a daily basis for HMG). This means taking blood samples to monitor your serum hormone levels; performing transvaginal ultrasounds (which are clearer than abdominal) to monitor the growth of the follicles, the quantity of follicles, and the size of your ovaries (see chapter 5 for ultrasound details); and taking vaginal smears to detect the quality of cervical mucus, also a marker for hormone levels. On your own, you should also be tracking your basal body temperature and the changes in your cervical mucus. The purpose of all this monitoring is to make sure that your ovaries are not enlarging, that your cervical mucus is the right consistency (CC can alter it), that intercourse is timed to coincide with ovulation, and that your ovaries are not forming cysts. You should not be on either CC or HMG unless you're being monitored.

What You Should Know About Multiple Pregnancies

In the 1950s, twins naturally occurred in 1 out of every 80 pregnancies. By the 1970s that number dropped to 1 out of every 100 pregnancies. Today, however, fertility drugs such as CC and

HMG have caused the incidence of multiple births to skyrocket: *Seven out of every 100 pregnancies are twins; 5 out of 1,000 pregnancies are triplets; 3 out of 1,000 pregnancies are quadruplets, and quintuplets—once exceedingly rare—occur in 1 of every 1,000 pregnancies.*

Carrying more than one fetus presents some special challenges that you need to stay on top of. Technically, blood tests and ultrasounds can you tell whether you're carrying twins in the second month of pregnancy. However, you may not know you're carrying more than one fetus until the second trimester because the pregnancy may seem quite routine. If you conceive through CC or HMG, make sure you let your obstetrician know (if he or she is not the same doctor who administered your drug therapy).

Early detection is important because the gestation period for a multiple birth is shorter than with a "*singleton.*" A single pregnancy is about 40 weeks long, but for twins the pregnancy tends to last only 37 weeks, while triplets are born at about 35 weeks. The more fetuses you're carrying, the shorter the gestation period. While gestation is shorter, the chance of premature labor is higher.

Carrying more than one child also means that your risks of low birth weights and cord problems are especially high. Some unique complications include *twin transfusion syndrome* (where one twin receives more nourishment and hence grows faster than the other), and the delivery of the second twin (which frequently requires a cesarean section). Pregnancy loss also increases, and the risks of developing all the other pregnancy problems such as *toxemia* (hypertension + water retention + protein in urine), gestational diabetes, and so on. Finally, if you have an existing red flag condition (such as Rh factor) that marks you as "high risk" from the outset, that condition can be exacerbated by multiple pregnancy, and you will go from a high-risk pregnancy to a very high risk pregnancy.

To manage a multiple pregnancy, you'll need to be under the care of an obstetrician and possibly a perinatologist (an obstetrician trained in high-risk pregnancies) if you have complications. In addition, you'll need to have a pediatrician who subspecializes in neonatal medicine, waiting in the wings for your first twin to be born. Your doctor should refer you to a pediatrician/neonatal specialist sometime in the second trimester, since you're likely to deliver prematurely. You will probably need several ultrasounds throughout the pregnancy. If you're over 35, you will also need to have an amniocentesis.

A Question of Cancer: Déjà Vu?

As discussed in the beginning of this chapter, many women's groups are questioning the long-term effects of "ovulation inducers" such as CC and HMG, claiming that the pharmaceutical and medical communities may be conducting an encore performance of DES, the Dalkon Shield (an IUD that caused pelvic inflammatory disease in users), and thalidomide (a drug widely distributed in the United Kingdom and Canada that caused horrific birth defects in the infants of users).

In January 1993, a study published in the *American Journal of Epidemiology* concluded that there was indeed an "associaton" between fertility drugs and ovarian cancer. This link was discovered accidentally, during an investigation of something else: whether oral contraceptive use and pregnancy *protected* women from ovarian cancer. The study found that women who ovulated less often were less likely to get ovarian cancer. Hence, women on hormonal contraceptives, women who were pregnant (you don't ovulate when you're pregnant), and women who breastfed (your cycle returns later when you breastfeed than if you were to bottle-feed) were more protected from ovarian cancer than women who were never pregnant or were never on hormonal contraceptives.

It was then found that infertile women who were never on hormonal contraceptives but who had been on fertility drugs *without success*, were at least three times more likely to develop ovarian cancer compared to the general female population (in the general population, the risk is 1 in 70). The study concluded that while the link was certainly alarming, much more research into the *long-term* effects of the drugs was needed before *any* kind of absolute conclusion could be drawn.

The media went crazy when this study came out. Numerous articles on the dangers of fertility drugs were published, while pharmaceutical companies sent out press releases documenting that the risks of fertility drugs and cancer were not proven and that fertility drugs were perfectly safe and effective.

When you're on these drugs, the amount of follicles you would normally produce in a year or even two years are being produced in a *couple of months*. Your ovaries are being worked overtime.

And, because it's an *undisputed* fact that women who give their ovaries a "break" from ovulation are less likely to develop ovarian cancer, it stands to reason that women who are overworking their ovaries are more *likely* to develop ovarian cancer. It's also an undisputed fact that women in the general population who never had children and were never on hormonal contraceptives are more at risk for ovarian cancer, too.

What this cancer risk means to you

The January 1993 study concluded that there were all kinds of data that needed to be computed into the ovarian cancer "risk profile" for fertility drug users. Without this data, conclusions about the absolute risks of these drugs cannot be drawn. The study noted, for example, that:

- Fertility drug users who conceived (regardless of length of pregnancy) were not at increased risk.

- Fertility drug users who had a history of past pregnancies (regardless of outcome) were not at increased risk.
- Fertility drug users who had a history of hormonal contraceptive use were not at increased risk.

The study also noted that none of the following factors was taken into account:

- Length of treatment
- Reason for treatment
- Strength of dosage
- Drugs or combination of drugs involved

It should also be noted that the study did *not* investigate how the following "known risk factors" affect fertility drug users:

- Family history of ovarian, breast, colon, or endometrial cancer (those with a family history of these cancers are more at risk)
- Obesity (obese women are more at risk)
- Diet (those consuming high fats are more at risk)
- Smoking (smokers are more at risk)
- Age (women ages 55–64 are more at risk)
- Exposure to toxins (this plays a role in risk)
- Menstrual history (women who are anovulatory to begin with have a greater risk)
- History of diabetes or hypertension (women with these histories are more at risk)
- Race (Caucasians and Northern Europeans are more at risk)
- Geographics (women living in urban centers are more at risk)

The bottom line is that without studying how the above data affect women taking fertility drugs, the cancer risk is, as the study concludes, "very tenuous."

What you should be concerned about

We didn't know the risks of DES, for example, until the children of DES users were old enough to reproduce. The children of DES users face the most profound risks of these drugs, not the DES mothers. So how will the *children* of fertility drug users be affected by the drugs when *they* want to reproduce? We have no idea. We suspect they will be more at risk for reproductive abnormalities (which won't be known until puberty in most cases); certain kinds of reproductive cancers; pregnancy complications, and birth defects.

To date, no increased risk of birth defects has been found among children born to fertility drug users. We won't know anything else until the babies born in the 1980s reach childbearing age, and that won't be until the twenty-first century.

Other Drugs That Induce Ovulation

Some women who are anovulatory will be given neither CC nor HMG. Instead, they may be offered one of the following drugs to compensate for a specific hormonal imbalance. In these cases they will not be taking an "ovulation inducer" but a hormone replacement. Therefore, risks such as hyperstimulation syndrome, ovarian enlargement, or cancer are not an issue.

Bromocriptine

Bromocriptine is the drug prescribed for *hyperprolactinemia,* which is discussed in chapter 5. Hyperprolactinemia means that you're producing too much prolactin, which inhibits estrogen production. High levels of prolactin are normal in pregnant and lactating women. For those who are not pregnant, alcohol consumption and antidepressant use can cause you to overproduce prolactin (see chapter 2).

Bromocriptine suppresses your hypothalamus, and hence suppresses prolactin. The most popular brand name of bromocriptine is Parlodel. This won't *cure* your hyperprolactinemia, but it will *control* it. The dosage is pretty low because bromocriptine is extremely potent. You'll start with about 2.5 milligrams per day, and eventually graduate to the same does three times a day. Once you get pregnant, you'll be taken off the drug immediately.

Risks and side effects
The side effects can be nasty: dizziness, nausea, nasal congestion, low blood pressure, and headaches. You'll usually experience the side effects at the beginning of your treatment, then find that they subside with time. This drug is considered safe, but it has only been in use for about a decade. So far, it hasn't been known to cause any birth defects, but it's still too new to yield any long-term statistics.

Before you start bromocriptine, you'll need a CAT (computerized axial tomography) scan to rule out the possibility of a benign pituitary tumor, which could be the source of your high prolactin levels. Other than that, there are no other conditions that prevent you from taking bromocriptine.

The odds

About 90% of women on bromocriptine will ovulate as long as they take it correctly; 65–85% of these women get pregnant. Multiple births and ectopic pregnancies do not occur with any more frequency than they do in the general population.

GnRH—Pump or Spray

In some cases, women have specific GnRH *deficiencies*, where their hypothalamus glands are not producing GnRH, which results in anovulation. Under these circumstances, you'll be put on clomiphene citrate first, and then move on to GnRH only if you don't respond to clomiphene citrate. Lutrepulse (a pump form) is the brand name for pure GnRH used for this purpose. A nasal spray called Synarel can also be used to remedy GnRH deficiencies. This drug has been abandoned by most fertility specialists. It was a hot item in the late 1980s and the early 1990s.

Operation Egg Retrieval

If you're undergoing IVF or GIFT or another ART procedure, and if you're ovulating regularly, you'll be prescribed HMG not so much to induce ovulation, but to stimulate the ovaries to produce several mature follicles. If you're not undergoing IVF, CC, and HMG may be used together. This is not a standard practice, but it is not necessarily more risky than HMG used alone. If your doctor suggests this combination, ask why it's being suggested over using HMG or CC alone. Almost all IVF programs place you on a GnRH analogue such as Lupron prior to the administration of CC or HMG.

In general, the side effects and risks of these drugs are the same for you as for an anovulatory woman. You must also make sure that the cause for your infertility (whether male factor or female factor) is investigated before you undergo any kind of ART procedure. When you're on these drugs, you will also require the same level of monitoring as an anovulatory woman, but you will *not* ovulate. Instead, your eggs will be *retrieved* through an egg retrieval procedure. The surgical procedures that follow greatly depend on the ART procedure you've chosen and are therefore discussed in the next chapter.

Drugs After Retrieval

If you're undergoing IVF-like procedures, you will begin HCG injections 35 hours before egg retrieval to keep your uterus primed and receptive for an embryo. After the embryo is put back inside you, you will either begin displaying the signs of early pregnancy, or you will begin to menstruate. The HMG cycle can begin immediately after your period is over, if you haven't conceived.

If you're not having an IVF-like procedure but are having your eggs retrieved so they can be put into a host uterus (because you are donating oocytes or cannot sustain a pregnancy for some reason), then you will also receive HCG prior to your retrieval surgery. You will either have your period induced by a progesterone suppository or will just stop all medication and shed your lining naturally. If the pregnancy hasn't established in the host uterus, you'll begin your treatment again after your period is finished.

Drugs Used in Male Fertility Therapy

When a man's levels of either FSH or LH (and consequently, low testosterone) are too low, it's a sign of a pituitary gland problem. This can be remedied with HMG, which is used to stimulate the seminiferous tubules and the Leydig cells (see chapter 4 for details).

For the majority of males taking fertility drugs, HMG (menotropins such as Pergonal) will be prescribed over clomiphene citrate, since clomiphene citrate has not been proven to be helpful for men. When menotropins are prescribed to men, they should only be taken if a man has undergone a full workup and has been diagnosed with a sperm-producing deficiency that is caused by *pituitary gland* failure. For example, if your sperm-producing problem is being caused by testicular failure (indicated through very high levels of FSH and LH), HMG is not an appropriate therapy.

HCG will also be taken in conjunction with HMG at an interval determined by your doctor. Generally, sperm production can be achieved only if HCG and HMG are used together rather than separately.

Side Effects

The only specific side effect reported with men on HMG is the development of enlarged breasts, known as *gynomastia*. This condition goes away once you stop treatment. As for headaches and nausea and the long list of side effects reported by women, there is no specific literature that cites whether these side effects are experienced only by women. No studies on cancer risks or other long-term risks have been done regarding male usage of HMG.

If you're taking HMG and HCG because of hypogonadotrophic hypogonadism (which may be caused by Kallmann's syndrome, discussed in chapter 4), HMG/HCG will be used to stimulate the onset of a puberty you never experienced. In this case, the drugs may cause what's known as "precocious puberty." This can be a dangerous situation in which your body suddenly goes into a wild, uncontrolled puberty, causing hormonal overload: huge increases in body hair, overgrowth of genitals, and a huge libido. If this happens, your HMG/HCG therapy will need to be stopped ASAP.

Other Drugs

Hyperprolactinemia can sometimes occur in men who are taking HMG. High prolactin levels in men are caused by a benign tumor in the pituitary gland, which will interfere with testosterone levels. This tumor can be removed, or *bromocriptine* may be prescribed to block prolactin secretions.

Finally, as mentioned in chapter 4, thyroid disorders can be common hormonal culprits that reduce sperm production. You'll be placed on levothyroxine sodium (thyroid replacement hormone), which you'll need to take daily. This drug may be prescribed after you're treated for hyperthyroidism (an overactive gland) or hypothyroidism (an underactive gland).

Fertility drugs may only first enter the treatment picture if you're embarking on an assisted reproductive technology procedure such as IVF or GIFT. All of these procedures are discussed in detail in the next chapter. Whatever the reason is for taking these powerful drugs, it's important that you make an informed decision. For many, the short-term outcome of a possible pregnancy outweighs the side effects and questionable long-term risks of the drugs. "I'd rather have a baby *now* than worry about possible cancer 20 years down the road" is a common attitude of fertility drug users, but it is not necessarily the *wisest* attitude. You owe it to yourself to learn and assess all the facts and risks before you decide.

8

A Work of ART

If you've found the cause of your infertility, and it cannot be reversed or treated successfully, you may be a candidate for assisted reproductive technology (ART), sometimes referred to as *assisted conception*. Couples with unexplained infertility are also ideal candidates for some of these procedures.

Until 1978, couples who couldn't conceive had two choices: adoption or childfree living. In 1978 the first "test-tube" baby, Louise Brown, was born. Since then, thousands of children have been born worldwide as a result of reproductive technologies that assist couples in the conception process. In the 1980s, the ethical implications of various assisted conception techniques were debated as critics argued over the moral issue of conceiving children in a laboratory. Yet essentially, these techniques are no more "immoral" than administering drugs that induce ovulation, correcting anatomical problems surgically, or *preventing* conception through contraceptive technologies. We now live in an era in which the term *family planning* has taken on a futuristic dimension. However, the technology of many of these procedures is by no means a perfected science. There is a high degree of trial and error involved, and a very high failure rate as a result. Many couples need to be assisted repeatedly before they have a successful pregnancy. Although ART is a wonderful option for couples who can't conceive, it is not a panacea to infertility. In fact, the ART process is difficult and stressful and requires a committed and emotionally stable couple.

Before you and your partner look into ART, it's important to examine all of the other alternatives in chapter 10. Seeking the services of a good counselor or therapist is often helpful when you're making this decision; it's difficult to be objective and realistic when you want a child so badly.

Although you may successfully conceive through the techniques discussed in this chapter, the risk of miscarriage is high and the rates of successful births are low. Ultimately, you need to weigh these risks against other options. You'll have to gauge whether you're strong enough to whether not only the disappointment and pain of infertility, but also the added anxiety of a high-risk pregnancy or the grief of potentially losing a pregnancy you worked so hard to achieve (see chapter 9).

This chapter discusses the range of ART procedures available to you as of 1995. These include in vitro fertilization (IVF), a.k.a. in vitro fertilization embryo transfer (IVF-ET), gamete intrafallopian transfers (GIFT) and zygote intrafallopian transfer (ZIFT), various hybrids of IVF and GIFT, micromanipulation techniques, such as injecting sperm into the egg (designed to improve the odds), techniques designed to improve sperm quality, and the use of donor "materials," which are sperm, uteri, and eggs. This chapter also provides guidelines for selecting various programs and donors; guidelines for making decisions about procedures, and, when possible, success rates and costs. (Many procedures are simply too new to yield any meaningful statistics. Costs may vary from clinic to clinic; state to state; and province to province.)

The procedures discussed in this chapter are very complicated and involve several steps. To *truly* grasp the nature of each procedure, a degree in molecular biology really helps! Since most of us can't boast this credential, I've provided you with as much information as a layperson can digest. If you're considering any of these procedures, a frank discussion with your specialist is a good idea. You may also want to consult the back of this book for a list of resources you can turn to for more information.

Who Should Manage Your ART Procedure?

First, get a fertility specialist! See chapters 1, 4, and 5 for more details. Second, unless you're unhappy with your current fertility specialist, be it a reproductive endocrinologist/gynecologist or a urologist/andrologist, whoever has handled your workups so far, and has diagnosed your fertility problem should manage your ART procedure. In some cases you may be referred to a separate clinic that specializes in the ART procedure you want done, or another doctor with other skills may be called in as a consultant. Any ART procedure usually involves embryologists who perform all the necessary lab work; however, you may never meet these specialists. Your specialist may also provide several ART services at his or her own clinic or through the hospital he or she is affiliated with.

If you've been recommended to an ART clinic and haven't yet had a workup, you MUST go through both the male and female workups first. See chapters 4, 5, and 6 for more details.

Selecting a Clinic

If you've been recommended to a clinic for any ART procedure that involves ovarian stimulation and egg retrieval, you need to ask a number of important questions before you make your selection. You should also review chapter 1.

1. *When did the clinic/program first perform the procedure I am undergoing?* The longer the facility has been in business, the better; newer clinics may have shorter waiting lists. Also keep in mind that some ART procedures are so new that "old" may not mean anything.
2. *How many babies have been born as a direct result of the facility's efforts?* Remember, pregnancy rates are not the same as the rate of live births. If you can, find out how many live multiple births resulted, too.
3. *How many ovarian stimulation/egg retrieval cycles has the facility managed successfully?* A good number to work with is roughly 25 cycles per month. The more cycles the facility manages, the more experience it has with dosage adjustment and surgical retrieval.
4. *How many embryo transfer procedures has the facility done?* Again, the more the better. Experience, experience, experience!
5. *How many pregnancies have resulted from the facility's efforts?* Compare pregnancy rates to the rates of live births.
6. *What is the facility's miscarriage rate?* This is important data if you can get it. (It should be made available to you.)
7. *How many doctors will be involved with my care?* What are their credentials?
8. *What are your candidate requirements?* Most programs have age limits.
9. *Is there a choice as to the number of embryos transferred?* (This is not relevant for GIFT.)
10. *Is embryo freezing available?* This will minimize the stress involved with a second attempt.
11. *How much time should I arrange to take off from work?* This is a crucial question that many couples forget to ask. You'll need to arrange for appropriate leaves of absences, arrange for proper rest, and reduce your social commitments,. Unless you're rested and healthy, the procedure won't have the optimum chances of success. If a clinic tells you that you won't need to take more than a day off work, this tells you that there is very little patient consideration at that particular facility.

IVF: In Vitro Fertilization

In vitro fertilization is also known as *in vitro fertilization-embryo transfer* (IVF-ET) because it involves culturing embryos in a laboratory and then transferring them back into your uterine cavity, bypassing the fallopian tubes completely. In many IVF clinics, you'll see the acronym IVF-ET instead of just IVF. The term *in vitro* means "in glass"; yet today, "in plastic" is more accurate. This is a process that combines using the fertility drugs discussed in chapter 7 (clomiphene citrate and human menopausal gonadotropin) to induce ovulation, removing those eggs via microsurgery and/or ultrasound, and then placing them in a plastic dish and fertilizing them with sperm.

Before you make your IVF plans, please remember that this process is expensive, stressful, and drawn out. (The process can cost up to $5,000 per attempt; in Canada, many IVF candidates are not covered by universal health care.) Also bear in mind that IVF usually requires at least two attempts for a successful outcome.

IVF was originally designed for couples with female factor infertility due to damaged fallopian tubes (see chapters 5 and 6). Today IVF is also used for assisting couples who have unexplained infertility, who have a variety of male factor infertility problems, such as poor sperm count or poor morphology (see chapter 4), and who are involved in various donor programs. *IVF is the "architecture" on which all ART procedures are based.*

The Stages of IVF

IVF is an involved four-step process. The first stage is ovarian stimulation via a GnRH analogue and then human menopausal gonadotropin (HMG). Even if you are ovulating regularly, you'll be placed on fertility drugs to stimulate the production of multiple follicles on your ovary. This increases your doctor's chances of obtaining a good, "fertilizable" egg. All of this is discussed in detail in chapter 7.

In the second stage, blood tests and ultrasound are performed, and eggs are collected. This is known as egg retrieval, oocyte pickup, or egg pickup. You'll be monitored daily. When your eggs are ripe, you'll undergo a procedure called endovaginal egg retrieval with the aid of ultrasound, where your doctor actually *retrieves* your eggs. (See the separate section on egg retrieval below.)

The third stage involves fertilizing the eggs in a lab. After the eggs have been fertilized by sperm, stage 4, *embryo transfer,* is the final step. Stage 4 involves transferring the embryos from the petri dish directly into the uterine cavity with the aid of a catheter.

The fertility drugs discussed in chapter 7 do tend to create chromosomally imperfect eggs, so you may need to have more than one cycle's worth of eggs retrieved before your doctor finds an acceptable one. When this happens, the egg is nurtured in the laboratory until it is mature enough to interact with the male partner's sperm. Any other good eggs retrieved might be fertilized and frozen for future embryo transfers, eliminating the need to go through ovarian stimulation and egg retrieval again. Embryo freezing is called *cryopreservation* (discussed in a separate section toward the end of this chapter).

You'll be given some notice about the timing of your egg retrieval. If your IVF procedure involves your partner's sperm, he'll need to abstain from ejaculation for about four days prior to delivering his semen sample to the lab. The semen sample isn't requested until enough satisfactory eggs are retrieved. Once the lab receives the semen sample, the sperm are carefully washed, which simulates the natural "capacitation" process sperm naturally go through when they swim upstream toward the egg. The sperm are also analyzed and the best sperm are selected for the dish. Then, the sperm are placed in the dish with the egg. If the sperm and egg fertilize, the embryo will be transferred to the uterus.

As discussed in chapter 7, if you're undergoing IVF, you'll not only receive injections of human chorionic gonadotropin (HCG) during the retrieval and fertilization stage, but your uterus will also be helped along by progesterone supplements after the embryo transfer to help make it as "embryo-friendly" as possible.

If the egg and sperm do not fertilize, you'll need to try again at the next cycle (if you choose to). In some cases, the failure of the sperm and egg to fertilize in the dish indicates other problems. Further tests may be necessary.

Egg retrieval

In the past, eggs were retrieved during a laparoscopy procedure. Today, most specialists will retrieve the eggs using an ultrasound-directed *needle aspiration* procedure. Needle aspiration does not require a general anesthetic, which translates into less stress for you.

The egg retrieval procedure involves a local anesthetic. Then, you'll undergo a similar procedure to a transvaginal ultrasound, except here, a needle aspirator is attached to the transducer. Using the picture on the screen to guide the transducer and needle aspirator, your doctor can reach your ovary and aspirate several follicles at once, retrieving them for use in an IVF-like procedure.

Oocyte culture and fertilization: An eggs-act science:

Once the eggs are retrieved, they're placed in fluid and counted and evaluated for maturity. This takes 2–3 hours. A semen sample, which will be collected and washed prior to egg retrieval, is incubated and then placed with the egg. The egg and sperm are then left alone for roughly 40 hours. If no fertilization takes place, other eggs retrieved during your cycle will be put together with new sperm from new samples. If no fertilization occurs and your egg supply is exhausted, you'll need to try again the next cycle. If the egg is fertilized, you'll go on to the final IVF stage, known as the embryo transfer or embryo replacement.

Embryo transfer

You'll report back to the hospital, where the fertilized eggs are transferred into your uterine cavity. Transferring the embryo back into the uterus is a far simpler procedure than retrieving the eggs. Your doctor will use a catheter to insert the embryo into your uterine cavity through your cervix. You will not require a local anesthetic, but you'll need to lie still for about 2–4 hours after the procedure. You'll then need to rest for the next 48 hours, getting out of bed as seldom as possible.

NOTE: *Roughly 10% of all embryos in IVF transfer well and actually implant themselves within the uterus.* This is a huge drawback that should make you question whether the stress of repeated IVF procedures is frankly, worth it. After the embryo transfer is done, you'll report to the clinic about two weeks later for a pregnancy test. If your test is negative, you'll need to decide whether you're going to repeat the process and *repeat the fee!* If a pregnancy doesn't occur after the embyro is transferred, you'll have to wait 3–4 cycles before trying another IVF cycle.

After the transfer, you'll receive hormone injections of HCG and may be placed on vaginal progesterone suppositories. As discussed in chapter 9, the progesterone supplements, many believe, will help keep the uterus receptive for the implantation and well primed for the early part of the pregnancy.

Is more than one embryo transferred at one time?

Generally, 3–4 embryos may be safely transferred into your uterine cavity. The shocking news is that even with this amount, the pregnancy rate hovers around 30–35%; the probability of twins with this amount is 12–15%, and there's a 2–4% chance of triplets. If you produce more than four embryos during one IVF cycle, the remaining embryos may be frozen (i.e. selected for cryopreservation) or may be used, with your permission, as donor eggs an issue discussed in the donor section further below.

Essentially, the more embryos that are transferred into the uterus, the greater the chance of multiple pregnancies. Most IVF-ET programs limit the amount of transferred embryos to three. The record for the greatest number of embryos transferred at one time is held by a British physician, who placed 11 embryos into a woman's uterine cavity. This was greatly criticized at the time for being risky and experimental.

Is there a way of minimizing the risk of genetic or chromosomal abnormalities in a developing embryo?

There is an experimental procedure known as an *embryo biopsy*. Here, one or two cells are taken from the developing embryo when it has divided into at least eight cells. The cells are examined for genetic and chromosomal abnormalities. If no abnormalities are found, the embryo is transferred. Otherwise, the embryo is discarded. Gender can also be determined with this procedure, but the sex can be withheld from the parents upon request.

What are the odds?

IVF does not carry encouraging success rates. First, bear in mind that only 55% of all pregnancies occurring in normal, fertile couples will result in a live birth. As for IVF, only 15–20% of all IVF pregnancies will result in a live birth.

Within 11–14 days after the procedure, a blood test can tell you whether a pregnancy has established itself. Although couples do conceive with IVF and do give birth to healthy children, the rate of miscarriage with an IVF pregnancy is greater than in the general population. Twenty-five to 30% of all IVF pregnancies will end in a first-trimester miscarriage, compared to the miscarriage rate of 15–20% in the general fertile population. Unfortunately, a woman's age does play a huge role in miscarriage statistics, which is why IVF carries rather dismal success rates after age 40. The miscarriage rate ranges between 45% and 60%.

Review chapter 9 for more details on pregnancy loss and the signs and symptoms of a first-trimester miscarriage. It's important to be prepared for these symptoms throughout the first trimester. The rates of miscarriage drop dramatically after 12 weeks, and at that point, the risk of pregnancy loss is the same with IVF pregnancies as in the general population.

How many IVF attempts should we endure?

If you haven't conceived after four *completed* IVF attempts, it's probably time to seek out alternatives (see chapter 10). However, many women may have one or more IVF cycles interrupted for a variety of reasons:

- *Poor follicular development.* This is often due to mistiming your hormone injections. When the follicle pickings are slim, you'll need to menstruate and start IVF at the next cycle.
- *Natural ovulation occurring prior to egg retrieval.* If your blood tests show that your lutenizing

hormone (LH) surge has occurred, indicating natural ovulation prior to the egg retrieval procedure, your IVF cycle will need to be discontinued and started again at the next cycle.

- *Too many follicles.* In some cases, your ovaries can become far too stimulated and produce so many follicles so early in the cycle that it's dangerous to your health. In this case, your doctor may stop the cycle and perhaps lower your fertility drug dosage during the next cycle.

- *Adverse reactions to the fertility drugs.* This is covered in chapter 7. There are a variety of adverse symptoms you may develop, such as pain and enlarged ovaries, that may necessitate stopping the IVF cycle before your eggs are retrieved.

Who's an IVF candidate?

IVF is obviously not for everyone, but there are some specific cases where it is an ideal option:

- *Women who have tubal blockages of some sort.* IVF in this case is tried *after* microsurgery, which can successfully "declog" a fallopian tube. After microsurgery, you'll try to conceive for another year or so before you seek out IVF. It's best to discuss the pitfalls and benefits of repeated microsurgery versus repeated IVF attempts. Keep in mind that many doctors will advise you to go directly to IVF instead of trying to repair badly damaged tubes. Once you've made your decision, you'll be required to go through a screening process by your selected IVF program/clinic, discussed below.

- *Women with endometriosis.* Again, your doctor will first try to treat your endometriosis through drug therapy and/or microsurgery (see chapter 6). If you don't respond and you still can't conceive after at least a year, you can seek out IVF.

- *Couples with immunological infertility.*

- *Men with low sperm counts.*

- *Men with poor morphology.*

- *Women who don't get pregnant with fertility drug treatment.*

- *Couples with unexplained fertility.*

Guidelines for making the IVF decision

1. *Are you familiar with the procedure, the costs involved, and the success rates?* If you can afford only one attempt, you might want to save your money and seek out an alternative. Most couples try once or twice. Most successes require at least a second attempt.

2. *Are you prepared to deal with the stress involved?* If you feel stressed now, wait until you begin IVF. You need to be in superb psychological "shape."

3. *Are you prepared to deal with a failed IVF attempt?* Remember, even if you're lucky enough to conceive, the miscarriage rates are high. Can you *really* handle losing this pregnancy? You might want to review chapter 9.

4. *Have you and your partner figured out how many attempts you're willing to go for?* Know your limits in advance, and know when to say "enough is enough."

Selecting an IVF program/clinic

Review IVF programs with either your reproductive endocrinologist/gynecologist or your andrologist/urologist. If this fails, refer to the resource list at the back of this book and contact some of the organizations for IVF clinic referrals. Then review the questions under the preceding section.

The screening process

Once you've made your decision on an IVF clinic, there is a screening process you'll need to undergo. For most programs you'll need to meet these basic requirements:

1. *Can you ovulate on your own?* In order for fertility drugs to work best you'll need to be able to ovulate on your own, and just have your ovulation "augmented" by the drugs.

2. *Do you have accessible ovaries?* If you have endometriosis growing all over your ovaries, scarring as a result of PID, or numerous fibroids blocking the way, your doctor will have a harder time getting to the eggs.

3. *How old are you?* Your fertility does decline as you age. Most programs have cutoff ages of about 40 but may give priority to women over 35.

4. *Have you had all your prepregnancy screenings done?* You'll need to be screened for certain conditions such as rubella. Check out chapter 1 for more information.

5. *Is the male partner's semen analysis normal?* It's hard to believe that some couples haven't checked this out before seeking out IVF, but it happens. In any event, if there are sperm problems, IVF won't work! Review chapter 4.

6. *Are you willing to go for a psychological workup?* You had better, because all programs recommend pretreatment counseling first. If you're not psychologically prepared IVF will do you no good.

7. *Can you afford it?* You may need to disclose your income and/or assets to the clinic. They won't attempt IVF if you can't pay for it.

Some Valid Questions

Q. *Is there a disproportionate number of male or female sexes with IVF babies?*

A. The boy/girl ratio is the same as in the general population.

Q. *Do the risks of birth defects increase with IVF babies?*

A. The birth-defect statistics are the same for IVF babies as in the general population.

Q. *Are there any special foods, herbs or exercises I can do to increase my chances of success?*

A. Unfortunately, there's nothing you can eat or do that will increase your chances of success. However, you should review the "Eating Habits" and "Exercise Habits" sections in chapter 2. There are some foods that can increase your chances of failure, and overexercising is the worst thing you can do while undergoing IVF.

Q. *Can I undergo IVF with donor eggs or donor sperm?*

A. Absolutely! IVF is an ideal solution if you need to mix and match reproductive material. See the separate section on donor insemination and oocyte donation.

GIFT: Gamete Intrafallopian Transfer

This is a very similar process to IVF, but it's about half as expensive and requires about a third of the time. The entire GIFT procedure takes about 40–60 minutes. GIFT carries slightly higher success rates than IVF, yielding a pregnancy rate of about 20–30%, but it also carries the same risks and stresses as IVF. The only differences are the following:

1. You need one good fallopian tube, normal semen, and a good postcoital test (PCT) result (see chapters 4 and 5). Usually, couples with unexplained infertility are the best candidates. (GIFT has been used on women with endometriosis or cervical mucus problems, couples with immunological infertility, or men with low sperm counts or poor motility, but without a good PCT test, the chances of success are much lower.)

2. Instead of fertilizing the eggs in a laboratory, the woman's mature eggs and her partner's washed sperm are mixed in a syringe together and inserted via laparoscopy right into her fallopian tube. A general anesthetic is necessary, which may make recovery uncomfortable. Then, you wait for nature to take its course.

What's Involved?

GIFT was developed in 1984 primarily for couples with "unexplained infertility" to facilitate a formal "meeting" of the sperm and egg. Like IVF, fertility drugs are used to stimulate the ovaries to produce multiple follicles. And, like IVF, the follicles are retrieved. Unlike IVF, there is no fertilization process that is done in a laboratory. Instead, roughly two hours prior to egg retrieval, a semen sample is delivered and put inside a centrifuge (that spinny thing) where it's washed and then placed in a test tube. The active sperm swim to the top of the test tube and are then placed inside a catheter. The mature egg is placed inside a separate catheter. Each catheter is then inserted into the fallopian tube via a laparoscopy procedure under a general anesthetic. Like an IVF procedure, a woman undergoing GIFT will need to rest quietly after the procedure and report for a pregnancy test roughly two weeks later. If pregnancy doesn't occur, a maximum of four GIFT cycles is recommended.

IVF versus GIFT

The downside of GIFT is that once the egg and sperm are transferred in the fallopian tube, there is a blackout period of roughly two weeks before you know if the procedure worked. With IVF, you know immediately after the procedure whether the embryos successfully transferred. Because of the waiting period involved with GIFT, a new procedure, called ZIFT, was developed, which brings the benefits of both GIFT and IVF together.

Some Valid Questions

Below are some common questions GIFT candidates ask, but you should still review the IVF questions above, too.

Q. *Would a GIFT cycle be interrupted for any reason the way an IVF cycle might?*
A. Again, like IVF, GIFT is dependent on fertility drugs for the procedure to work. The same conditions (such as poor follicle development) that would cause your doctor to stop an IVF cycle would cause him or her to stop your GIFT cycle, too.

Q. *Will the laparoscopy procedure involved with GIFT damage my ovaries or my tubes?*
A. Laparoscopy is a fairly exact science. It's highly unlikely that a skilled laparoscopist will nick you. That's why the word *skill* is so important when you interview your surgeon.

Q. *Is there a higher rate of ectopic pregnancy with GIFT?*

A. Slightly. Statistics are awfully tricky when it comes to figuring this out, but essentially, if you compare the GIFT population to the general population, the rates of ectopic pregnancies are slightly higher, but that's because the sperm and egg are placed directly inside the fallopian tube. Review chapter 9 for more information on ectopic pregnancy.

Q. *What's the rate of multiple pregnancy with GIFT?*

A. Current studies suggest that up to 30% of all GIFT pregnancies are multiple. This happens when more than one egg is transferred into the fallopian tube.

Q. *What happens to extra eggs retrieved in a GIFT cycle?*

A. That depends on you. You can freeze the eggs to be used in a future GIFT cycle or a future IVF cycle, or you can donate the eggs. You'll be offered all of these options.

Q. *How long should I abstain from sex after the procedure?*

A. Anywhere from 5–7 days of abstinence after a GIFT procedure is recommended.

Zygote Intrafallopian Transfer (ZIFT)

ZIFT is what you get when you cross GIFT with IVF. ZIFT eliminates that blackout period associated with GIFT. Essentially, ZIFT is exactly the same procedure as GIFT except that instead of transferring raw egg and sperm into the fallopian tube, the egg and sperm make a pit stop in a petri dish, where they are fertilized but not cultured into embryos. Instead, the fertilized egg and sperm are transferred in their "undivided" state, which is called a zygote. To refresh your memory, raw or untampered egg and sperm are gametes; fertilized egg and sperm prior to cellular division are zygotes; fertilized egg and sperm that have begun cellular division are embryos.

In a ZIFT procedure, the transfer of the sperm and egg is done 18–52 hours after egg retrieval, so the egg and sperm can fertilize. Like IVF, either laparoscopy or an ultrasound-guided transvaginal procedure is used to transfer the zygotes into the fallopian tube.

Why choose ZIFT?

If you are a GIFT candidate but can't handle the waiting involved with the procedure, then ZIFT may be an option. However, ZIFT is a much newer procedure than GIFT, and is not yet offered by many infertility clinics. The ZIFT success rates are considered similar to GIFT, but it is thought to be a better procedure than GIFT for couples facing male factor and immunological infertility. In severe cases of male factor infertility, the pregnancy rate after ZIFT is roughly 28%, and the rate of ectopic pregnancy is not any higher than with other ART procedures.

Tubal Embryo Transfer (TET)

Tubal embryo transfer (TET) is identical to ZIFT except that it transfers a 48-hour-old embryo into the fallopian tubes instead of a zygote. This procedure is too new to yield any meaningful success rates, and like ZIFT, not too many clinics practice TET.

Intravaginal Culture

Intravaginal culture is a new procedure developed in France. It works exactly like any IVF procedure, except the egg and sperm are put inside the vagina instead of inside the fallopian tube or a petri dish, with a diaphragm put in place to "hold them there." Then, if the egg is fertilized, it is transferred IVF style directly into the uterus. The vagina is used as the incubator in this case because it's cheaper than a petri dish. The procedure is too new to yield any meaningful statistics yet.

Cryopreservation/Frozen Embryo Transfer (FET)

Whenever you produce extra embryos in an IVF procedure, you'll be asked if you'd like to freeze them for future IVF attempts. Cryopreservation will reduce much of the expense and anxiety involved with a future IVF attempt, since you will not require ovarian stimulation or egg retrieval. Instead, on your second attempt, your cycle will be monitored only to gauge when your endometrium is receptive to the embryo. Then, you'll have a frozen embryo thawed in the lab and transferred into the uterine cavity. The most successful freezing of a human embryo is when it's done at the "pronuclear" stage, which is anywhere from the first to the sixteenth cellular division. These embryos can be stored for up to three years. Sixty to 80% of all embryos are viable once they're thawed.

Artificial Insemination by Partner

In the past, artificial insemination by partner was known as AIH—artificial insemination by husband. In a politically correct era, the word *husband* has been changed to *partner*. However, the appropriate acronym is not AIP, but simply AI. Currently, clinical circles have once again reworded artificial insemination to "therapeutic insemination." (TI) When a donor is involved, the term "therapeutic donor insemination" (TDI) is used. Since this book is designed for the lay public, I'll use the more familiar terms, AI and DI.

AI is an option for cervical mucus problems, low sperm count, poor motility, or sperm antibodies. AI is also an option for psychological problems that affect male sexual performance (such as impotence), and for physical problems such as obesity coupled with a small penis, which can also affect male sexual performance. Here, the male partner's sperm is collected semen-analysis style (see chapter 4), washed, and then injected by syringe either very high into the vagina (this carries only a 13% success rate) or directly into the uterus (this carries a 10–25% success rate). This is done only after you've tried to treat your infertility with other means. When a woman undergoes insemination with a stranger's sperm or sperm that is not her own partner's, AI becomes *DI—donor insemination*—discussed separately below. Generally, DI is an ideal option for couples with untreatable male factor infertility (resulting in azoospermia), or for single women or lesbian couples desiring children.

This is not a difficult procedure at all, but any woman undergoing AI must be able to ovulate; be clear of any luteal phase defects in order to have an "embryo-friendly" uterus; have a good set of fallopian tubes; and have no other pelvic abnormalities.

AI Recipes

There are three ways to artificially inseminate. Homologous insemination (a.k.a. "cup insemination," or "the cup") is when the male partner's semen is washed, separated to improve motility, and placed in a diaphragmlike cup at the cervix during ovulation. In order to place washed sperm in the cup, you'll need to be inseminated at your clinic or doctor's office. However, in many cases doctors may show their patients how to insert the cup properly so that between sperm washes, couples can do the procedure with fresh, unwashed sperm.

Intracervical insemination (ICI) is a little more involved. Here, a GIFT-like spinning of the semen (via centrifuge) is done to collect the best sperm. It is then placed in a catheter, which is used to pass the semen directly into the cervical canal. For each ICI attempt, you'll need to be inseminated at your clinic or doctor's office. Many couples will combine ICI with the cup to improve the odds between ICI attempts.

Unfortunately, the success rates for both the cup and ICI are low; so far these procedures haven't proved to be any more successful than spontaneous conception for oligospermic (low-sperm count) men.

Intrauterine insemination (IUI)

This is probably a more familiar acronym. As discussed, IUI yields far better results (10–25%) than ICI or the cup as long as the insemination is timed properly. Just before ovulation, the semen is washed and spun with a sample of the male partner's blood, which creates a pellet of sperm with no semen. The dead or immotile sperm are then separated from the good sperm, placed in a catheter, and placed directly into the uterus. Sometimes fertility drugs are combined with an IUI procedure.

ART for Men

When IVF-like procedures fail because of the inability of the sperm and egg to fertilize naturally, because of either immunological infertility or various male factor problems, there are now some science fiction–like procedures that can help fertilization occur. These procedures are known as micromanipulation. Critics of this new technology argue that this infertility treatment goes "too far" and removes the the crucial "natural selection" process that all human reproduction depends on.

Micromanipulation of Gametes

This procedure is used to help facilitate a successful IVF or ZIFT. Washed or capacitated sperm are literally injected into the retrieved egg with a tiny needle. This injection procedure is carefully done under a microscope and is called microinjection. The moral issue is this: Are we injecting defective sperm into the egg, increasing the chances of a defective embryo, pregnancy, or fetus? We don't know the answer yet.

Intracytoplasmic Sperm Injection (ICSI)

Similar to micromanipulation, this newer hybrid involves injecting *one single sperm* directly into the egg. So far ICSI is yielding good results, with a pregnancy rate of roughly 30%. ICSI is an excellent ART procedure for subfertile men with poor sperm counts, poor morphology, or poor motility. Most clinics require at least two standard IVF attempts before they will perform ICSI. The same "natural selection" issues are raised with ICSI, however.

Zona Pellucida Drilling (a.k.a. Zona Drilling)

In BiologySpeak, the *zona pellucida* is a protective layer of cells that surround the female egg. If you imagine a hard-boiled egg, the zona pellucida is the shell and egg white, while the portion carrying all the genetic material is the yolk. The scientist's job is to drill through the shell and egg white so that the sperm can be directly injected into the yolk. Meanwhile, in a basic microinjection procedure, the sperm is injected into the egg white and left on its own to make it to the you.

Zona drilling and partial zona dissection (PZD) use the microinjection procedure to make a gap in the zona pellucida either mechanically or by applying a solvent from a microneedle. In theory, sperm with low motility or a low count could fertilize the egg when placed in the drilled hole.

The problem with zona drilling is that there is greater risk of more than one sperm fertilizing the egg, which can lead to some freakish fertilization problems (known as *polyspermia*). Critics of zona drilling argue that the zona pellucida serves an important purpose in guarding against this. And again, are we introducing defective sperm into the egg?

Microsurgical Epididymal Sperm Aspiration (MESA)

MESA doesn't carry the same questionable morality as microinjection or zona drilling. MESA is really a rescue mission using microsurgical techniques. The money is in the bank, you can count it and see it, you just can't withdraw it. As discussed in chapter 4, when there is an absence or defect of the vas deferens, a man may have perfectly normal sperm that are obstructed. This is an entirely different problem than a testicular defect. In this case, the sperm are alive and well but are trapped inside the epididymis.

With MESA, the sperm can be rescued from the epididydmis and brought together with the female partner's egg through IVF or ICSI. For a woman, the IVF procedure is the same as for any other woman undergoing these procedures. But for the male partner, instead of delivering a sperm sample, he'll undergo a microsurgical procedure under a general anesthetic in which his sperm are aspirated from his epididydmis and transferred into the woman. MESA is recommended for men with a congenital (present from birth) absence of the vas deferens, failed vasectomy reversal, or other problems due to obstruction of the vas deferens.

If MESA cannot be done, an *alloplastic spermatocele* can be inserted. This is a device that can be implanted into the the working part of the epididymis. This implant acts like a pouch that collects sperm, which can be aspirated by a needle and artificially inseminated into the female partner. Occasionally, the epididymis is missing or damaged. Sperm can now be extracted directly from the testes for use in an ICSI procedure.

Nonsurgical Techniques That Improve Sperm

Whenever a couple undergoes an IVF-like procedure or any of the artificial insemination procedures discussed below, there are several techniques designed to improve the odds by improving sperm quality.

Washing

Washing is a now a standard procedure in any IVF/GIFT-like procedure, regardless of sperm count. The sperm are separated from the semen by being spun in a centrifuge. This removes the proteins and enzymes that protect the sperm's head, enabling it to enter the petri dish or fallopian tube fully capacitated, a process that would occur if the sperm were allowed to naturally swim up the reproductive tract. The technique involved in washing and separating sperm to improve motility is highly technical and is therefore too complicated for the average person to truly comprehend. However, despite the complexities involved in the lab work, the only thing a male patient needs to do is deliver a sperm sample. If you're curious about the whole sperm washing process, your doctor will be happy to draw you a diagram.

Filtering

Filtering is reserved for men undergoing ART because they've had poor semen analyses in all areas. Here, fine spun-glass fibers are put into a syringe with the sperm, where they are required to pass through the fibers. In theory, the dead sperm should stick to the filter and not make it through. This is a highly experimental procedure with unconfirmed success rates.

Improving volume

When there is more semen than sperm, getting past the cervix may be a problem, since most sperm is in the first few squirts of ejaculate. Men with poor sperm volume or viscosity are encouraged to withdraw from the vagina just after ejaculation starts. Or they may withdraw prior to ejaculation, collect their semen, and drop it off to a lab for an artificial insemination procedure.

If the problem is more sperm than semen, then the sperm will never make it to the cervix. In this case, the semen is collected and washed and artificially inseminated.

Donor Procedures

Today, both men and women donate reproductive material to help couples and singles biologically parent a child. Until fairly recently, donor insemination (DI) was the only ART procedure that came to mind when one thought of a "donor." However, surrogate mothers are also considered donors, donating either their eggs and wombs (the traditional surrogate mother), or thier wombs only (known as host uterus, where the egg comes from a woman other than the host). Many women also donate just their eggs, known as oocyte donation. The bottom line is that many children are born from the reproductive materials of three people rather than two: donor sperm, donor oocytes, and donor womb. Although this makes for nightmarish family law legislation, today donor procedures are proving to be satisfying solutions for thousands of couples who desire children.

The donor procedures themselves are not in any way different from the acronym soup I've covered so far: IVF, GIFT, ZIFT, or AI can all be used to mix and match genetic materials. The pressing physiological issues surrounding donor procedures involve *appropriate screening*.

As for the emotional and moral issues involved with donor procedures, this section will touch on some of these issues, but to be perfectly boring and frank, the decision-making process is highly individualized and depends on your cultural, religious/spiritual beliefs, and emotional health. I'll do my "guidelines thing" that may certainly help you to look at certain questions and issues, but I will not be able to give you a profile of the "ideal" donor procedure candidate, because there is no such thing.

Donor Insemination

If you haven't read chapter 4, go back and do it now. It's important that you have an accurate diagnosis of untreatable male infertility before you make this decision.

DI is an option for couples with untreatable male infertility, for single women desiring children, or for lesbian couples desiring children. The costs range between $250 and $500. DI usually doesn't have to involve fertility drugs unless the woman does not ovulate regularly or is undergoing a more involved procedure. For example, DI can involve any of the artificial insemination procedures discussed above, or in cases where a woman has tubal or other structural problems, DI can be combined with IVF or even a host uterus.

Safe DI

I urge you *not* to try self-insemination at home with a turkey baster! In order to have successful DI, you must have "safe DI," and make sure that you select a program that screens its donors not only for STDs such as HIV or hepatitis B, but also for a range of genetic problems that could endanger a pregnancy. Even if you select your own donor and know him well, it's not possible for a complete screening to be done unless you involve a qualified lab. Compiling your own "questionnaire," for example, just won't cut it! Of course, not all sperm banks or DI programs practice appropriate screening procedures. You'll need to assume the "buyer beware" mentality while hunting for a DI clinic.

Guidelines for finding safe DI programs

1. Find out how long your DI clinic/sperm bank has been screening for HIV. Then, ask how old the "oldest" sample is. Any sample taken before 1990 still may be tainted with HIV, the AIDS virus.

2. Ask for a list of all the conditions the donor is screened for prior to delivering the sample. Again, HIV isn't the only infection you'll want to avoid. The donor should be free of all chlamydia, mycoplasma, gonorrhea, herpes, hepatitis B, and so on. The donor should also be free of genetic problems, such as Tay-Sachs disease or sickle cell anemia.

3. Ask about the screening process. First, all clinics should be using at least Red Cross guidelines for screening donors, but good clinics are even stricter. These guidelines include asking about sexual habits and histories that go back to 1977 (i.e. "Have you slept with prostitutes, other men, etc., since 1977?"). Second, as of 1986, most donors should have been tested at the time of their deposits. Their semen should have been frozen, and then the donors should have been retested in 180 days for HIV. If they were still negative, their semen was used. But HIV can take up to six months to show up in an AIDS test. Select a donor program that screens in six-month intervals to be safe.

4. Ask if the clinic keeps permanent records of donors (confidential), which can be made available to a couple or offspring if requested. Will nonidentifying information on the donor be released to adult offspring if requested? For example, if two DI adults meet from the same program, will they be able to find out if they have the same father?

5. Is the sperm fresh or frozen? Until 1986, most sperm banks preferred to use fresh semen over frozen, because fresh yielded higher success rates. Today only frozen semen should be used to reduce the risk of HIV infection. Fresh semen is *not* acceptable.

6. Does your clinic/program enforce a limit as to how many offspring one donor can father? The American Fertility Society recommends 10 pregnancies per donor as a maximum. This number is based on population density, lowering the outcome/probability of two half siblings meeting and marrying.

Once you've selected your program . . .

Once you've chosen a donor clinic/program that you're comfortable with, you'll discuss with an assigned counselor what kind of physical features you require, genetic lineage, and so on. When that process is complete, you'll be able to choose the AI procedure that you're most comfortable with: IUI, ICI, or even the cup, but most clinics will do either ICI or IUI. At the time of ovulation, the insemination will take place in the clinic. Prior to insemination, it's crucial that the woman undergoes a complete physical and pelvic exam to screen for other barriers to fertility, or for problems that may endanger a pregnancy. Once the insemination is done via ICI or IUI, a cervical cap or nonabsorbent sponge will be placed at the cervix to keep the sperm in place. You may require several attempts before a pregnancy establishes.

The success rates of DI are usually higher than AI because both participants are usually completely fertile. Meanwhile, couples seeking AI are doing so to compensate for an already established fertility problem. Success rates range between 40% and 80%. Because of the stress involved, a woman's otherwise healthy cycles may become irregular, but this will usually correct itself without the use of fertility drugs.

Surrogate Parenting

Surrogacy is DI in reverse. It is an option when the female partner cannot ovulate and cannot carry a fetus. Here, a fertile surrogate mother is artificially inseminated with the male partner's sperm. This will produce a child that has the male's and surrogate's genes.

Finding a suitable surrogate is a little more complicated than finding a suitable male donor because there is far more involvement with the surrogate, who will complete the pregnancy and give birth to the child. However, the process involves finding a program that screens surrogates for sexually transmitted diseases (STDs), HIV, and a range of genetic problems. It also involves selecting a surrogate who has genetic features similar to those of the female partner's.

Surrogate parenting is a custom that goes back to the Old Testament. The first case of surrogacy involved Sarah and Abraham. The infertile Sarah (who probably just needed some clomiphene citrate) "offered up" her handmaid, Hagar, to her husband Abraham. With Abraham's sperm, Hagar conceived and bore him a son, Ishmael. (Unfortunately, Sarah got very jealous later on and cast out Hagar into the wilderness. Then, she herself conceived a child at the age of 100—that's really pushing back the biological clock!)

Surrogate mothers can be found through a donor clinic or program, or by contacting family law practitioners who specialize in adoptions (see chapter 10). Surrogacy is considered an offshoot of adoption. To date, there have been well under 10,000 surrogate arrangements in North America, but it's predicted to become a booming business in the very near future. The lawyer will draw up a contract between the infertile couple and the surrogate mother, addressing issues such as miscarriage (will she try again?), and so on. If the surrogate changes her mind, the contract is no guarantee that the courts will take your side. You'll also need to pay a fee to the surrogate, which may average from $10,000 to $100,000.

Fortunately, there are a few offshoots of surrogacy that enable women to biologically mother a child, by borrowing only the uterus and not the eggs.

Surrogate Gestational Carrier

This is an option for women with structural or medical problems that prevent them from carrying a fetus to term. In this case, an IVF procedure is performed with the woman's own eggs and her partner's sperm. The embryo is transferred into another woman's uterus, who will than carry the baby to term. The child, therefore, is the genetic offspring of the infertile couple and does not biologically belong to the carrier in any way. In order to do this, a woman must be able to ovulate on her own, and the male partner must be fertile.

Often, a relative of the woman is selected—usually a sister or mother—who can share the pregnancy experience with her. The success rate is about the same as IVF, but might work better in this case because the gestational carrier may have a more receptive uterus.

Donor Uterus (a.k.a. Host Uterus or Embryo Transfer)

When the male partner is fertile but the woman has an irreversible problem that does not respond to treatment, a donor uterus is considered. A woman will need to have a healthy uterus for this and be able to sustain a pregnancy. The male partner's sperm is inseminated into a donor uterus. When a pregnancy results, the woman's uterus is "prepped" for a pregnancy with fertility drugs, and the embryo is transferred from the donor uterus into the woman's own uterus, where she will continue the pregnancy and give birth to a child who has the donor's genes and her own partner's genes. This is not yet a very successful procedure; there's a high rate of miscarriage or failure for the embryo to implant.

Oocyte (Egg) Donation

As discussed in the IVF section, whenever a woman is having her eggs retrieved for an IVF or GIFT-like procedure, she may be asked about cryopreservation (embryo freezing) or oocyte donation if her cycle has yielded more follicles than can be used in a single procedure. Cryopreservation will preserve extra embryos for a woman's own use in future procedures, or for use in a procedure where donor embryos are required.

As in any DI procedure, anyone undergoing a procedure with donor eggs will need to make sure that the donor is screened for all of the conditions previously discussed, such as HIV and other STDs. There are some unique conditions that apply to the oocyte screening process:

1. All donors should be of legal age.
2. Younger donors tend to provide better pickings. Any woman over 34 years old should have her age revealed to the recipient so that appropriate testing during pregnancy can be offered.
3. Previous pregnancies by the donor is an asset.
4. The donor should be screened for any X chromosome linked genetic disorder.
5. All risk factors for HIV infection should be taken into consideration (intravenous drug use, etc.). If the donor falls into a known risk factor group but tests negative for HIV, she should still be disqualified.
6. The donor should be screened for all conditions that would create a high-risk pregnancy, such as Rh incompatibility.
7. The recipient should be offered a choice of having the donor's eggs fertilized and frozen, and then having the donor recalled for HIV testing six months later. If she still tests negative, the embryos may be used.

To date, egg freezing has a greater risk of causing chromosomal damage to the egg because the freezing stops cellular division, which may interfere with future fertilization. Most procedures that require donor eggs use "fresh eggs" instead of frozen.

Who can benefit from donor eggs?

Any woman suffering from poor or absent ovulatory function can receive donor eggs. These women may be anovulatory and do not respond to fertility drugs, or they may be suffering from premature ovarian failure as a result of early menopause or cancer therapy. Whatever the reason for their ovarian failure, as long as they have a viable uterus and can sustain a pregnancy, they can undergo IVF or GIFT (if they have good tubes) with donor eggs and their partner's sperm. Unfortunately, women pregnant with donor eggs have a higher rate of pregnancy loss and a higher implantation failure rate. This is believed to be caused by an overall reduced capacity to maintain a pregnancy in the first place.

Women over 40 are classic candidates for donor eggs. Generally, the rate of infertility in women over 40 is 30% greater than in younger women, while the miscarriage rate in women over 40 is about 50% using ART. Therefore, success rates using traditional ART methods are less than 10%. Because of egg donation, these dismal ART statistics are changing. It's found that eggs from younger women have an equal rate of success in ART procedures as the ART statistics in the under-40 age groups.

Other women who can benefit from oocyte donation are those who carry X-linked genetic diseases; those whose eggs cannot be fertilized despite several IVF attempts; those who have inaccessible ovaries as a result of endometriosis or PID, for example; and those who suffer from repeated miscarriages despite treatment.

The most progress with oocyte donation has been made in treating women with premature ovarian failure, which occurs in 1–3% of the female population. In this group, ART with egg donation is the most successful treatment for infertility, with success rates as high as 50%. The pregnancies that result are usually normal, allowing the mothers to breastfeed after birth.

What does oocyte donation involve?

Any woman who decides to donate her eggs will be placed on fertility drugs to stimulate multiple follicles on her ovaries. The eggs are then retrieved using the same procedure discussed in the IVF section. Meanwhile, the recipient of the eggs will have her uterus prepped with appropriate hormonal therapy so that she can sustain the pregnancy. If the recipient ovulates naturally, she will have her cycle controlled by artificial hormones that will interrupt the natural cycle. An endometrial biopsy will be done on the recipient prior to embryo transfer to make sure that the endometrium is the right thickness to sustain an implantation.

When the oocytes are retrieved, they will be mixed with the male partner's sperm and transferred into the recipient in an IVF, GIFT, ZIFT, or other IVF-like procedure.

Who is an appropriate donor?

The donors are usually infertility patients who agree to donation, freezing their eggs for future use. Often, donors are close relatives or friends of the recipient. Essentially, any premenopausal woman is an appropriate candidate. Once she is selected (or has agreed to donate), a full physical, STD screening, and psychiatric workup are required. The donor also needs to provide her full medical history and a family medical history. Oocyte donors can be a sister or other relative of the recipient. Some centers advise against asking a relative or friend to donate because the decision is often made out of debt or out of guilt.

Anonymous donors allow the recipient to select from a larger pool of eggs. Again, many anonymous donors are already undergoing IVF, but some may agree to do it in exchange for payment. In general, IVF patients are seen as ideal anonymous donors.

A Word About Disclosure

If you give birth to a child who results from one or more donors, you and your partner will need to discuss whether you will disclose your child's true identity to family members, friends, and most important, to the child. This is a highly individual choice. Whatever you do, don't make the decision without weighing all the pros and cons. For instance, would telling unreceptive family members damage the child's relationship with them, or your relationship with them? Seek out other couples who have children of donors and see what their disclosure process involved. Ultimately, there is no right or wrong answer regarding disclosure, just open- and closed-minded people. There are numerous books that can help a child accept his or her beginnings. One can compare this new controversy over disclosure to issues concerning *adoption* disclosure. Twenty years ago, many people thought it was wrong to tell an adopted child that he or she was in fact adopted. Today, almost all children who are adopted are informed that their parents are *not* their biological parents. You might want to take the Pennsylvania Reproductive Associates Infertility Survey (PRAIS) © in Figure 10. A low score indicates that you have a preference for disclosure.

Obviously, the complexity and stress involved with any ART procedure is monumental. This makes a failed attempt or even a miscarriage all the more traumatic. Options to biological parenting may become more appealing if you have a bad ART experience, and decisions about your parenting future may become clearer as you go through the ART haul. In any event, chapters 9 and 10 should be read by any ART candidate to prepare for a pregnancy loss, and to prepare for other alternatives, including adoption and childfree living.

Pennsylvania Reproductive Associates Infertility Survey (PRAIS) ©

Author's note: A low score indicates a preference for disclosure

Name _____ Age _____ Occupation _____

Gender: ___ male   ___ female
Religion: ___ Catholic   ___ Protestant   ___ Jewish   ___ Other
Marital Status: ___ Married   ___ Single   ___ Divorced   ___ Separated   ___ Widowed
Experience with infertility: ___ myself ___ friend   ___ family   ___ none

This survey looks at people's opinions about different kinds of infertility treatments for married couples. Please take a few minutes to answer as openly as possible. Circle the number of the response that most closely represents your opinion. It is important that you answer each question and leave no blanks. Listed below are brief explanations of less familiar medical terminology:

Donor sperm: The sperm of another man is used to fertilize the egg of a woman whose husband is infertile.

Donor egg: Another woman's egg is fertilized with the sperm of the husband whose wife is infertile and wife carries the pregnancy.

In Vitro Fertilization (IVF): When the couple's egg and sperm are collected medically and allowed to fertilize in a laboratory; the fertilized egg (embryo) is then placed in the wife's body.

Gestational Carrier: When a woman is medically unable to carry a baby in her womb, her egg is collected and fertilized with her husband's sperm in a laboratory. The fertilized egg (embryo) is carried by another woman (gestational carrier), and at birth the baby is given to its biological parents.

	Strongly Agree	Agree	Disagree	Strongly Disagree
1. Parents should tell their child that they used donor sperm to conceive that child	1	①	3	4
2. Men who permit their wives to be artificially inseminated will have mixed feelings about their children	1	2	3	④
3. I believe that gestational carrier programs should be illegal	①	2	3	④
4. I do not consider egg donation a sin	①	2	3	4
5. No matter how much a woman will love a child born to her using a donor egg, she will never feel it is truly hers	1	2	3	④
6. If I used donor sperm, I would tell my friends	1	2	3	④
7. I would feel dirty having an unknown man's sperm in my body (males: answer as if you were a female)	1	②	3	4
8. If a man is sterile, he is less virile	1	2	3	④
9. I would be willing to be a sperm/egg donor	①	2	3	4
10. Children born of donor sperm or eggs are the same as any other children	①	2	3	4
11. The woman who conceived a child through donor insemination will love him/her more that her husband will	1	2	③	4
12. Legally, the man who donated the sperm is the father	①	2	3	4
13. Parents should tell their children they were conceived through in vitro fertilization	1	②	3	4

	1	2	3	4
14. Men who donate sperm have a moral responsibility toward that child	1	2	3	(4)
15. I would feel OK about my husband donating sperm (males: answer as if you were a female)	1	(2)	3	(4)
16. Parenthood is given to those who are truly deserving	(1)	2	3	(4)
17. Couples who use donor egg or sperm to have a baby are asking for trouble	1	2	(3)	(4)
18. If I used donor eggs or sperm, I would tell my family	1	2	(3)	4
19. Parents should tell their child that they used a donor egg to conceive the child	1	(2)	3	4
20. I would feel OK about my wife donating eggs (females: answer as if you were a male)	1	2	(3)	4
21. The man or woman who donates sperm or eggs should have legal rights as the child's genetic parent	1	2	3	(4)
22. I would choose adoption before I would choose to use a donor	1	2	3	(4)
23. A woman who uses donor sperm is hurting her husband, even though he agrees	1	2	(3)	4
24. No one should know that the child was conceived by use of a donor except the involved couple and the medical personnel	(1)	2	3	4
25. Couples who use IVF are being selfish	1	2	3	(4)
26. Feelings about having a child conceived by use of donor will always bother the couple	1	2	(3)	4
27. I do not consider donor insemination a sin	(1)	2	3	4
28. No matter how much a man will love a child born to his wife through donor sperm, he will never feel that it is truly his	1	2	(3)	4
29. If I used donor eggs, I would tell my friends	1	2	3	(4)
30. Couples who use donors are being selfish	1	2	3	(4)
31. Using a gestational carrier is like playing with fire	1	(2)	(3)	4
32. Making a child belongs to a married couple—not to medical science	1	2	3	(4)
33. Parents should tell their children they used a gestational carrier	1	(2)	3	4
34. Women who use donor eggs will have mixed feelings about their children	1	(2)	(3)	4
35. Being a gestational carrier places tremendous stress on the carrier's marriage	1	(2)	3	4
36. I believe gestational carrier programs are unethical	1	2	(3)	4
37. Using a donor egg or sperm is committing adultery	1	2	3	(4)

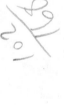

PRAIS © is reprinted with permission of Pennsylvania Reproductive Associates, 1994.

Figure 10.

9

Pregnancy Loss

I wish I didn't need to write this chapter but, unfortunately, many couples who have struggled with fertility have a higher risk of losing the pregnancy. Repeated pregnancy loss is considered to be another form of infertility, even though initial conception may not have been a problem.

This chapter discusses the types of problems that can occur during the first trimester and early second trimester of a pregnancy and can lead to pregnancy loss. Issues surrounding *repeated miscarriage*, which refers to having three or more miscarriages in a row (i.e., consecutive miscarriages) before 20 weeks are discussed in a separate section. Under these circumstances, it's important that both partners undergo a full workup to eliminate problems that may be contributing to the pregnancy loss.

While factors leading to pregnancy loss can occur later in a pregnancy, resulting in premature birth in the third trimester or even in a stillbirth at term, this chapter will *not* discuss pregnancy loss issues beyond the early second trimester. You see, the risk of pregnancy complications dramatically *drops* as the pregnancy progresses. For couples who conceived through an ART procedure (see chapter 8) or with fertility drugs (see chapter 7), the risk of pregnancy loss beyond the early second trimester is no greater than that of the general pregnant population. (At that point you can graduate to my book *The Pregnancy Sourcebook*, which will discuss everything you need to know throughout the entire course of pregnancy and the postpartum phases.)

Finally, this chapter also includes information on a unique pregnancy loss issue known as vanishing twin syndrome. This is essentially the loss of one twin while the other develops normally. Many women who have had fertility drugs may be susceptible to this problem, which has been largely ignored by the medical community until the last decade or so.

What Are the Odds?

If you haven't had any ART procedures and are pregnant solely as a result of fertility drugs, such as clomiphene citrate or human menopausal gonadotropin (see chapter 7), you have a greater risk of having a multiple pregnancy, but your risk of miscarriage is not any higher than that faced by the general population: 1 in 6. If you've already had more than two miscarriages in a row, please review the section entitled "Repeated Miscarriage." You should not attempt conception again before a complete workup is done.

What you *will* need to do is to make sure your levels of human chorionic gonadotropin (HCG) are checked regularly in the first two months of pregnancy (high levels are signs of multiple pregnancy). You should also request an alphafetoprotein (AFP) screening and an ultrasound as early on as you can, which can also confirm or rule out a multiple pregnancy. If you're pregnant as a result of fertility drugs such as bromocriptine or gonadotropin-releasing hormone (GnRH) (see chapter 7), your risk of a multiple pregnancy or a miscarriage is no greater than that faced by the general population.

If you've had any kind of tubal repair surgery, your risk of an ectopic pregnancy is greater than that of the general population because your tubes may have scarred as a result of the repair procedure. You'll need to review the symptoms of ectopic pregnancy discussed in this chapter. Seek medical attention if you notice any of them.

If you're pregnant as a result of artificial insemination, your pregnancy is no more risky than a routine pregnancy (except for the multiple pregnancy issue if you had fertility drugs). If your pregnancy resulted from in vitro fertilization (IVF), gamete intrafallopian transfer (GIFT), intrauterine insemination (IUI), or any similar procedure (including microinjection), you not only have a higher risk of miscarrying, but you also have the multiple pregnancy issue to rule out. Anything transferred directly into your fallopian tubes will make you more susceptible to an ectopic pregnancy. However, if your ART procedure involved transfer of gametes or embryo directly into your uterus, your risk of ectopic pregnancy is nil. You should definitely be seeing an obstetrician trained in reproductive endocrinology once your pregnancy is established, however, regardless of which ART you had.

Problems in the First Trimester

When something goes wrong at this stage, it has to do with the pregnancy not "taking." This usually means two things: a miscarriage (bleeding and cramping are the main symptoms) or an ectopic pregnancy (sharp, abdominal cramping or searing pain on one side—it depends on the tube). Often, women don't even *realize* they're pregnant until they experience a first-trimester problem like this. But these problems are common even in the general pregnant population. Ectopic pregnancies were considered a less common occurrence until about five years ago, when the results of sexually transmitted diseases (STDs), pelvic inflammatory disease (PID) and assisted reproductive technology started to factor into the childbearing population. If you've had PID, (and well over one million North American women do), you are at a higher risk of suffering an ectopic pregnancy. If you're walking around with chlamydia or gonorrhea, you're also at risk. *Studies estimate that as many as 50% of all women between the ages of 18 and 30 have chlamydia and don't know it.* This is why it's important to be screened for STDs prior to conception.

As for miscarriage, one in six pregnancies in the general population ends in miscarriage, *and 75% of these miscarriages occur before 12 weeks.* The risk of a miscarriage also increases with age. If you're over 35 and pregnant as a result of an IVF-like procedure, your risk of miscarrying is quite high.

Bleeding

Bleeding during pregnancy isn't normal, but it's not *unusual* either. Nor does it mean that a miscarriage is imminent. Some women may continue to have scant periods during this trimester. In fact, in the general population, some women don't realize they're pregnant until about three months into the pregnancy because of this. Although menstrual cycle changes usually won't be noticed until about weeks 4 and 5, you can spot as early as seven days after conception. This is known as *implantation bleeding* and is a normal vaginal spotting caused by the formation of new blood vessels, but it's rarely experienced.

It's crucial to note whether any *pain* accompanies your staining or bleeding. Staining or bleeding with no pain is better news than staining or bleeding with cramps. Nevertheless, bleeding or spotting of *any* kind during this stage should be reported immediately to avoid any risk.

The most dangerous kind of bleeding at this point is heavy bleeding. The definition of heavy bleeding means that you need to change your pads about every hour. Other danger signs to watch out for are *additional symptoms* accompanying the bleeding, such as cramps, pain in the abdomen, fever, weakness, and vomiting. If the blood has clumps of tissue in it, this is also a bad sign. If this is the case, save your pad. Just stick your whole pad, clumps and all, in a baggie and save it for the doctor to look at. Put the baggie in the refrigerator until you take it to the doctor. If this isn't done (particularly if left overnight), the tissue degenerates and smells, and a pathology exam cannot be done. The clumps may be important clues to what's going on. You may also notice an unusual odor accompanying the bleeding. If light bleeding or spotting continues for more than three days, this is another, less obvious danger sign.

Does your bleeding *always* mean that you're losing the pregnancy? No. Vaginal bleeding can occur if you have an infection of some kind, lesions, a polyp. or a fibroid.

Regardless of why you're bleeding, you'll need to follow the emergency procedures outlined in this chapter. You'll then need to undergo an internal pelvic exam, a blood test to see if your level of HCG is normal, and an ultrasound.

Miscarriage

There are several reasons why a miscarriage occurs. Some studies indicate that about 60% of all first-time, first-trimester miscarriages occur because of genetic abnormalities. It's your body's way of doing its own "genetic engineering," expelling malformed fetuses. More than 90% of women who miscarry once will go on to have successful pregnancies.

Symptoms
Heavy bleeding and cramping anywhere between the end of the second month to the end of the third month are classic signs that you're in the process of miscarrying. Cramps without any bleeding are also a danger sign that you're miscarrying. The bleeding can be heavy enough to soak several pads in an hour, or may be "manageable" and more like a heavy period. You may also be experiencing *unbearable* cramping, that renders you incapacitated. Sometimes you can pass clots, which are dark red clumps that look like small pieces of raw beef liver. Sometimes you may pass grayish or pink tissue. A miscarriage can also be taking place if you have persistent, light bleeding and more mild cramping at this stage.

If you suspect a miscarriage...
In the United States, if you're under the care of a private physician, you will usually have a chance to consult with your doctor about your symptoms over the phone (most of them are on

24-hour pagers). Depending on your situation, your doctor may be able to evaluate what's going on just by what you're describing over the phone, ask you to come into his or her office for an ultrasound, which can determine the status of the pregnancy, or ask you to meet him or her at the hospital. If you *are* miscarrying, sometimes a dilation and currettage (D & C) procedure can be scheduled at a convenient time for you, rather than as an "emergency" procedure. In fact, many doctors in private practice can actually do a better job of evaluating the problem in their offices than in a hospital emergency room.

For American women in less exclusive health care plans, as well as Canadian women (whose physicians do not have appropriate ultrasound equipment in their offices), you will need to inform your doctors' offices of your symptoms and *go directly to the hospital (or your birthing facility)*. Ask your doctor(s) to meet you there. Someone will take care of you when you get to the hospital or birthing facility.

Once you're in the hospital, your doctor will be able to tell whether you're indeed miscarrying, and what stage the miscarriage is in. He or she will do a gentle pelvic exam and/or ultrasound. You might be sent home with a list of instructions and told to wait it out, which is often the only thing to do. Sometimes it takes several hours for a miscarriage to run its course. Or, depending on what's going on, you might need to stay and have an emergency D & C procedure.

When you miscarry before 20 weeks, it's actually called a *spontaneous abortion*. However, there are several kinds of spontaneous abortions. Staying in the hospital or going home will depend on what kind of miscarriage you're experiencing, what stage it's in, and so on.

- *Threatened abortion.* Your cervix is still closed and holding everything in securely, but you're having cramps, bleeding, or staining. Your doctor will examine you and check the fetal heartbeat. You may also need an ultrasound. Then you'll be ordered to bed. In some cases, the bleeding will stop and the pregnancy will continue normally. Sometimes you might miscarry anyway because of unsalvageable problems, such as severe genetic deformities.

- *Inevitable abortion.* In this case, nature has already taken its course, and the process of miscarriage has started. Bleeding is heavy, cramps increase, and the cervix begins to dilate. You may wind up expelling everything while it's still intact: the fetus, amniotic sac, and placenta, accompanied by a lot of blood. This is the most traumatic kind of first-trimester miscarriage because you'll need to *save* what you've just expelled. Sometimes you'll have to retrieve these things from the toilet. If you're going through this, try not to be alone. Call a friend or make sure your partner is with you. If your doctor suspects an *inevitable abortion*, abnormal bleeding is usually heavy enough to warrant a D & C before any tissue passes out on its own. However, if a D & C is not done, the pregnancy tissue would come out on its own eventually. You'll need to save what you expelled in case your doctor wants to perform tests. But in general, it's difficult to determine the cause of an abortion by examining or testing expelled tissue.

- *Incomplete abortion.* This is when you're not naturally expelling all of the uterine contents. Some, but not all, pregnancy tissue has been spontaneously expelled. Usually what remains are fragments of the placenta. This needs to be corrected with a D & C procedure, which will clean out the uterus and help it to heal. You'll still need to save part of what comes out, but it will just look like clumpy pieces of blood. You may be sent home from emergency only to have to go back into the hospital a couple of days later for the D & C.

- *Complete abortion.* This is when all pregnancy tissue is passed spontaneously. You will be sent home and will *slowly* expel everything by steadily bleeding. This will feel like a miserable period, but everything will come out in time. You still may need a D & C anyway just to clean out little bits of tissue left behind, but this usually isn't necessary. The bleeding can actually go on for days until you're finally done. In this case, save anything that looks like pregnancy tissue and show it to your doctor.

- *Missed Abortion.* The fetus dies in the uterus but doesn't come out. You may not have symptoms for quite some time. This is when you just lightly spot and can mistake it for the "good bleeding." In this situation, all of your pregnancy symptoms will gradually disappear, and you obviously won't progress at all. This condition is frequently diagnosed during a routine exam, and the fetal heartbeat can no longer be heard. Treatment depends on the duration of the pregnancy.

Will it happen to me?

Again, the risk of miscarriage increases with age. The risk is about 10% for women in their 20s, and skyrockets to 50% for women in their mid-40s. This means that a significant portion of thirtysomething pregnancies will end this way. There are all kinds of reasons why you might be miscarrying, but most women who miscarry either once or twice do go on to have normal pregnancies and deliveries. The odds of having a miscarriage tend to increase exponentially with each *recurrent* miscarriage. In general, with no past history of miscarriage, your odds of having one are about 12%. After one miscarriage, the odds remain at about 12%. After two miscarriages in a row, the odds of having another are 27%; after three in a row, the odds jump up to 36%; and after four miscarriages in a row, the odds skyrocket to 60%. Because of this, it's important to STOP trying after two consecutive miscarriages to be evaluated for factors causing pregnancy loss.

After one miscarriage, the expelled contents will be examined for any clear signs of why the miscarriage happened. Usually, a fetus is "self-terminating" because it wasn't developing properly. If this is the case, then there usually isn't a known cause for your miscarriage. You'll need to wait anywhere from 3 to 6 months after a miscarriage before you try again, or resume fertility treatments. Choose an appropriate barrier method to prevent conception during this period.

One cause cited for miscarriage are an *incompetent cervix*. Some women are just born with an incompetent cervix, but it can be weakened by a previous miscarriage or therapeutic abortion. Other causes are chromosomal abnormalities; infections; hypertension or diabetes; and progesterone deficiency.

Possible causes of miscarriage at this stage involve hormonal deficiencies that interfere with fetal development, uterine structural problems, genetic error, and blood incompatibility.

It's helpful to seek out other women who have gone through pregnancy loss as well. There are several support groups for women who have miscarried once or twice.

Some women may have more severe reactions to pregnancy loss than others. These reactions may include sleep disturbances, psychosomatic illness, worsening of a previous illness (such as asthma), irritability, and avoiding social contact (particularly friends with children or friends who are pregnant). A good therapist can help you work through some of these feelings, which are valid and common under these circumstances.

Ectopic Pregnancy (a.k.a. Tubal Pregnancy)

An ectopic pregnancy occurs when the embryo never makes it to the uterus and starts to develop in the fallopian tube. Sometimes the embryo can even develop on the ovary or in the abdomen; in this case, it's known as an *abdominal pregnancy*, which *has* been known to go to term (but that's *Guinness Book* material). If an ectopic pregnancy goes undetected, it strains the tube, which isn't designed to expand like the uterus. Then, 6 to 8 weeks after conception, the embryo will cause severe abdominal pain and possible vaginal bleeding. If the pain is more pronounced on one side, this is a textbook symptom of ectopic pregnancy.

Ectopic pregnancies are very dangerous. If your tube ruptures, you could suffer severe internal bleeding, which is a life-threatening situation. Common symptoms of ectopic pregnancy are sharp abdominal cramps or pains on one side. The pains may start out as a dull ache that gets more severe with time. Neck pains and shoulder pains are also common. You may also have a menstrual type of bleeding along with the pain, but the pain is the most *obvious* sign.

The problem with ectopic pregnancies in the general population is that often women don't realize they're pregnant until they have one. If you've been seeking fertility treatment, you'll typically have a pregnancy test before the start of each new cycle. There are also other high-risk groups for ectopic pregnancies that will help to alert you to the possibility.

- Women who wore intrauterine devices (IUDs).
- Women with a history of PID.
- Women with a history of pelvic surgery (scarring may block the tube and prevent the egg from leaving).
- Women with a history of ectopic pregnancy.
- Women pregnant as a result of assisted conception techniques, where gametes or embryos have been injected into their fallopian tubes.
- Women with endometriosis (see chapter 6).

If you have symptoms of ectopic pregnancy or suspect it, follow the instructions outlined in the emergency procedures section below. Your doctor will check your HCG levels (a pregnancy test), and an ultrasound will be done to see the condition of the uterus and fallopian tubes. Once the ectopic pregnancy is confirmed, you will need *emergency surgery and a skilled surgeon*. The surgery involves removing the embryo from your fallopian tube. This is delicate surgery, and you'll want someone who is capable of saving your fallopian tube if possible. Sometimes this isn't possible, and your fallopian tube will need to be removed (known as *salpingectomy*). Depending on the progression of the pregnancy, you may need one ovary removed as well (known as an *oophorectomy*). You'll then need to recuperate for at least a week from surgery. After surgery, you'll need to repeat some blood tests to make sure no embryonic tissue is left. Usually, women go on to have normal pregnancies afterward. You'll need to have at least two natural periods before you try to conceive again. If you have only one fallopian tube or one ovary, the remaining tube or ovary will "pick up the slack" and you'll ovulate regularly.

Although the incidence of ectopic pregnancy has increased, the fatalities from it have *decreased*. This is largely due to major innovations in laparoscopy. Many surgeons can safely remove the embryo, preserving the tube, through *laparoscopy* (operating with a thin telescopic instrument with the aid of a video camera), instead of doing more invasive abdominal surgery. In addition, some ectopic pregnancies can be diagnosed *before* there are any symptoms simply by checking levels of progesterone and HCG. Transvaginal ultrasound and uterine curettage are also helpful diagnostic tools.

How common is it?

In 1995, ectopic pregnancies, once a fairly rare occurrence, are considered fairly common. Between 1970 and 1987, the incidence of ectopic pregnancies rose from 18,000 to 88,000, a *huge* increase, now accounting for 1.5% of all pregnancies in the United States alone. The consequences of an ectopic pregnancy may be upsetting. In women who aren't fortunate enough to have the ectopic diagnosed early, over half will not conceive again. Meanwhile, 10–15% of all ectopic sufferers will have a repeat episode.

What researchers *do* know is that many of the lifestyle habits discussed in chapter 2 seem to play a large role in ectopic pregnancy risk. Women who smoke less than 10 cigarettes a day have been found in some studies to have a 40% greater risk of ectopic pregnancy. Women who smoke more than 30 cigarettes a day are *five times* more likely to have an ectopic pregnancy. Nicotine affects the mobility of the fallopian tubes. This may delay implantation because the tube contractions (which move the embryo along into the uterus) are affected by estrogen levels, which smoking seems to reduce. In addition, smokers can't fight off infections as effectively as nonsmokers, which puts them more at risk to certain STDs, which can lead to PID. Again, the increase in chlamydia and PID directly corresponds to the rise in ectopic pregnancies. One British study revealed that 76% of women who had ectopic pregnancies were also found to have antibodies for chlamydia.

Emergency Procedures

What's the definition of an *emergency* at this stage? Heavy bleeding, severe pain (cramps or abdominal), sudden, severe vomiting that doesn't seem to be related to your morning sickness, loss of consciousness, and, in later trimesters, symptoms of early labor. If you're taken by surprise by the symptoms discussed in the two sections above and feel they are severe, immediately call your fertility specialist, gynecologist, or primary care physician's office. If it's during business hours, ask the receptionist or answering service what hospital your practices at (they all will be affiliated with a hospital). Have the receptionist inform the doctor that you will meet him or her there and that you're leaving *now! Then, get yourself to the emergency unit of that hospital ASAP.* If you can't drive yourself or find someone to take you, by all means *call 911 and request an ambulance.* If it's after hours, there should be a recorded message at your doctor's office that gives out an *emergency number* and the *address* of the hospital he or she is affiliated with. If you're well enough to go on your own, have someone (friend, mother, spouse, neighbor) call that emergency number and arrange for the doctor to meet you at the hospital. If you're going by ambulance, the ambulance staff will call for you.

If for some reason you can't get a hold of any doctor, and he or she does not have prerecorded emergency instructions, get yourself to the emergency unit of *any* hospital ASAP, either on your own or by ambulance. Once you're there and being looked after, the hospital will sort everything out and find the doctor and appropriate hospital for you. Never wait for the doctor to call you back. Also review the section "If you suspect a miscarriage" above.

Problems in the Second Trimester

The risk of ectopic pregnancy is almost nil beyond the twelfth week of pregnancy, while the risk of miscarriage really dramatically drops by this stage. Yet those women in a "high risk" category will continue to worry about the pregnancy beyond the first trimester. Because of this, I've provided information on the kinds of problems to look out for beyond 12 weeks, even though your "danger time" technically has most likely passed.

When something goes wrong in the pregnancy at this point, it usually has to do with either *your* health—be it infection, structural problem, or injury—that might trigger a miscarriage or premature labor, or a problem with the *placenta*, which may trigger the same things.

Bleeding

This time, light or spotty bleeding is often caused by an increasingly sensitive cervix, which may be irritated in an internal exam or Pap smear (if you need one for any reason), or sexual intercourse. Notify your doctor immediately about the bleeding. Heavier bleeding at this stage can also be caused by either a low-lying placenta (*placenta previa*) or the premature separation of the placenta (*abruptio placenta*), but these problems are more commonly found in the third trimester. Bleeding can also be a sign, once again, that you're losing the pregnancy, or that you're experiencing premature labor.

Late Miscarriage

Between the third month and twentieth week of pregnancy, a spontaneous abortion is known as a late miscarriage. The symptoms are similar to the first trimester miscarriage variations. In many cases, a condition known as an incompetent cervix is responsible. This is when the cervix dilates prematurely and cannot "hold in" the fetus. This condition is also known as a weak cervix. For the most part, the causes of an incompetent cervix are unknown, but trauma to the cervix as a result of infection, for example, can trigger premature dilation.

Incompetent cervices are also more common if you're a DES daughter due to a possible malformation of the cervix. See chapter 1 for more information on DES daughters. If an incompetent cervix is caught early enough, as may be the case if you've had repeated miscarriages at this stage, the cervix can be stitched up and the pregnancy can be resumed. Then, at around 38 weeks or prior to labor, the stitches can be removed and a normal vaginal birth can take place. Some stitching techniques are permanent, however, and a cesarean section is necessary.

If the miscarriage is inevitable and can't be prevented, a D & C can be performed up until the 20th week. A miscarriage after 20 weeks is no longer a miscarriage and graduates to either a premature birth or, in unfortunate cases, a stillbirth. Under these circumstances, you'll need to follow the steps outlined above under "Emergency Procedures."

Premature Labor

Premature labor is characterized by contractions accompanied by vaginal bleeding, vaginal discharge, or even a vaginal pressure anywhere from the 20th week to the 37th week. Premature rupture of the membranes (the amniotic sac) occurs in 20–30% of all premature deliveries and is a sign that something is wrong as well. Other symptoms of premature labor are menstrual-like cramps with possible diarrhea, nausea or indigestion, lower back pain, and all the other symptoms of labor.

Between 5% and 8% of all deliveries are premature. The health of the premature newborn depends greatly on how premature the delivery is, what kind of neonatal care is available, the weight of the newborn, and how developed the newborn is. Babies born before 25 weeks (weighing slightly more than 2 pounds) have about a 50% chance of surviving, *assuming* that they're receiving appropriate treatment in a neonatal unit. When the newborn weighs 3 pounds or more, his or her survival jumps to about 95%.

What causes premature labor at this stage?
The causes of premature labor at this stage are unknown, but there *are* some factors that can trigger it:
- Poor general health: cigarette smoking and inadequate nutrition can increase your risk of premature labor.
- Diabetes and/or thyroid problems that have not been treated appropriately.
- Cocaine use.

- Syphilis (review chapter 1 on STD screening).
- Placental problems.
- Physical trauma, such as a car accident or a bad fall.

What should you do?

This is an *emergency situation* and can be treated with medications to postpone the labor. As soon as you begin contractions, contact your doctor immediately. You'll need to go directly to your birthing facility or the emergency room at the nearest hospital. Follow the "Emergency Procedures" outlined above. If you're successful in halting the contractions with medication, you may be put on strict bed rest for the duration of the pregnancy.

Depending on how severe the situation is, your doctor may decide to proceed with delivery. If your membranes have ruptured or you're having vaginal bleeding, there is no way you can stop the labor; you'll need to go ahead and deliver. If, however, you have ruptured your membranes but are experiencing *neither* contractions *nor* any vaginal bleeding, the pregnancy may be "saved" with medications and continue to term. This happens in about 25% of the cases. In the worst-case scenario, the baby is delivered prematurely and treated in a neonatal unit. Premature labor is more commonly a third trimester problem, however.

Vanishing Twin Syndrome

Vanishing Twin Syndrome used to be considered more rare than it is now thought to be. Again, with the popularity of fertility drugs and assisted conception techniques, multiple pregnancies are on the rise. As many as 80% of all twin pregnancies (which occur in about 7 out of every 100 pregnancies) will experience this phenomenon, in which the pregnancy starts out as a multiple pregnancy, but only one fetus actually develops.

Symptoms of vanishing twin syndrome are actually similar to symptoms of miscarriage: vaginal bleeding, cramps, or decreased hormone levels, but then a healthy fetus may be discovered during the ultrasound. More often though, there are no symptoms and the second twin is reabsorbed by the body, while remnants of the placenta and membrane may be delivered at the birth of the surviving twin. In some cases, remnants of a second placenta during delivery may be the only clue that a twin has "vanished."

This syndrome probably would not even have been discovered if it weren't for ultrasound technology. With ultrasound, two fetuses may be detected as early as the first trimester, and then, in the second trimester, you may be told that one has "vanished." This can be traumatic for many women, and is an experience that is not well documented or openly discussed. As ultrasound technology improves and more twin pregnancies are diagnosed in the first trimester, perhaps we will learn more about the reasons behind this phenomenon.

Repeated Miscarriage

If you've miscarried more than twice in a row prior to 20 weeks, you're prone to what's known in lay terminology as "repeated miscarriages." (Clinical terms for this are *habitual abortion* or *recurrent fetal loss*.) This *is* considered a form of infertility, but in my opinion, labeling "repeated miscarriage" as "infertility"—meaning inability to conceive is inaccurate! Repeated miscarriages have to do with an inability to complete the pregnancy. This is truly a different kind of problem than not *becoming* pregnant to begin with. Nevertheless, women who suffer from repeated miscarriages will need to undergo a battery of tests under the care of an "infertility specialist"—a reproductive endocrinologist/gynecologist.

If you have no history of full-term pregnancies, then you suffer from *primary repeated miscarriage*. If you've had one child or even a stillbirth at term, you have *secondary repeated miscarriage*. Tests include an *endometrial biopsy* (see chapter 5) and a *hysterosalpingogram* (where a dye is injected into your fallopian tubes, checking *not* for blockages, as discussed in chapter 5, but for uterine abnormalities). In most cases of repeated miscarriage, the cause is found; in a few cases, nothing is ever discovered as the definitive cause. Women who have suffered as many as six or seven miscarriages, however, can go on to have a successful pregnancy.

One cause of miscarriage has to do with untreated bacterial infections, such as mycoplasma. As discussed in chapter 1, if left untreated, mycoplasma can lead to an inflamed endometrium (endometritis), which can interfere with the embryo implanting. Another cause of some miscarriages is the effect of certain toxins, discussed in chapter 2, that include anesthetic gases (that's why the consent form for a surgical procedure tells you about a risk of miscarriage). Exposure to lead and mercury are also causes, but usually these toxins are discovered before a *second* miscarriage.

Other causes cited for repeated miscarriage include genetic problems, structural problems involving the uterus or cervix (such as an incompetent cervix, discussed above), luteal phase defects (discussed below), diabetes, and thyroid disease (if it's not treated promptly).

Luteal Phase Defects

Some doctors believe that a significant number of repeated first-trimester miscarriages are caused by a progesterone deficiency; others don't subscribe to this theory at all, even though there is strong evidence to support it.

Once your ovary spits out a follicle, the empty shell turns into a corpus luteum. If you imagine a single pea pod, the pea is the follicle which will become the egg, while the pod is what will turn into a corpus luteum, which should produce progesterone once the embryo implants. Human chorionic gonadotropin (HCG), secreted from the developing placenta, stimulates the corpus luteum to make progesterone. As the placenta matures at about 7 weeks, it takes over progesterone production. However, if the corpus luteum is not functioning properly and is therefore not making adequate amounts of progesterone, you will miscarry. Hormonal tests that include an endometrial biopsy will confirm whether you have this type of luteal phase defect.

The treatment is simple, involving daily dosages of natural progesterone in vaginal suppository form during the luteal phase of the menstrual cycle. Then, if conception occurs, progesterone suppositories are prescribed daily for the first 12 weeks of pregnancy. The average dosage is 50 milligrams of progesterone twice a day, but some women will be given a stronger prescription of 100 milligrams of progesterone taken 2 or even 3 times a day. Some doctors will also prescribe clomiphene citrate prior to conception, which will increase the amount of progesterone throughout the early stages of pregnancy. The progesterone suppositories are given once the pregnancy is established. Clomiphene citrate is also associated with lower incidences of miscarriage. Progesterone supplements are successful about 80% of the time in averting another miscarriage.

Repeated miscarriages can be caused by a scrambled LH (luteinizing hormone) surge. Normally, the LH surge occurs just prior to ovulation, but in some women, the surge can take place at the beginning of the cycle (common in women suffering from polycystic ovarian syndrome (PCO). The treatment is to be placed on a urofollitropin (pure FSH) or a GnRH analogue (see chapter 7 for details). This is still in the experimental stages, but studies show that this treatment is promising.

Immunological Factors

Between 20% and 25% of all repeated miscarriages are due to immunological problems. The woman's immune system causes her body to reject the fetus as foreign tissue for the same reason transplant patients reject organs. In this case, the mother's body is rejecting the father's antigens (a.k.a. paternal antigens) that make up the developing fetus. This problem can often be solved through either passive immunization (injecting the mother with the father's antibodies prior to conception) or active immunization (injecting white blood cells from both the mother and father into the mother's body before conception). In either case, the point of this treatment is for the mother's body to get used to his cells so that they recognize the fetus later on as friendly. Some clinics report about a 70% success rate using this method. Usually, giving the mother only paternal white blood cells yields the best results.

Other immunological causes involve women who produce antibodies that indirectly cause clotting in blood vessels that lead to the developing fetus. The fetus is deprived of nutrients and dies in utero, which triggers a miscarriage. There are no definitive treatments for this, although some clinics are looking into combining asprin, corticosteroids, or anticoagulants such as *heparin*.

Less Common Causes

About 15% of all repeated miscarriages are caused by a uterine structural problem, where tissue interferes with fetal development. This is usually correctable with surgery, depending on the severity of the defect. About 3% of repeated miscarriages are caused by an "incompetent cervix." This problem leads to second trimester miscarriages and can be prevented by stitching up the cervix. While about 5% of repeated miscarriages (as opposed to single episodes) are caused by chromosomal abnormalities, this is not a "correctable" problem, but a "luck of the draw" cause. It is also the cause of most first-time miscarriages, which occur once in six normal pregnancies. In this case, couples need to keep trying until they strike a good mix of chromosomes.

How Many Miscarriages in a Row Should We Endure?

After two miscarriages, you should stop trying and go for diagnostic tests to see *why* you're miscarrying. Often, the reasons are unknown and you'll go on to have a successful third pregnancy. Even after two miscarriages, there's a 70% chance that your third pregnancy will be fine. But if a reason does turn up, it may be easy to fix, and finding the cause at this point will prevent further trauma to you. Keep in mind, though, that one or two miscarriages do not make you infertile and are generally *not* precursors to future problems.

When Should You Cut Your Losses?

There is no right answer to this question. For some couples, one miscarriage or ectopic pregnancy is enough for them to seek alternatives to natural conception. For other couples, natural conception is still a goal even after seven or eight miscarriages. The point is not how many pregnancy losses you *should* endure, but how many you *can* endure. Of course, it's always important to find out, if possible, what the cause of your pregnancy loss was. There are often logical explanations behind the loss, and they *can* be treated.

While no one can prevent you from trying to conceive as many times as you like, the following is a list of guidelines to help you decide what "enough" means to you, personally. This list was compiled with the help of several couples who have been through pregnancy loss.

How Do You Define "Enough"?

1. What was the nature of your loss: miscarriage or ectopic pregnancy? Repeat ectopic pregnancies are rare if you're clear of STDs and had your tube salvaged or removed. A second miscarriage in a row is statistically less common than a successful pregnancy following a second miscarriage.

2. How many miscarriages have you had? Again, if no cause for your second miscarriage was found, you're statistically more likely to have a successful pregnancy on your third try than a third miscarriage. And with every idiopathic (i.e., no cause found) miscarriage, no matter how many in a row, the odds of having a successful pregnancy on the next try are greater than another miscarriage.

3. If a cause was cited, is it treatable? If a cause has been found for your pregnancy loss or losses, but there's no way of treating it, trying again will not make the problem go away. In fact, it will put you at risk for another loss. On the other hand, if there is treatment available and your doctor feels your chances of carrying to term on the next try are better than half, you may regret not trying again.

4. How old are you? The risk of miscarriage increases with age, while the risk of Down's syndrome increases as well. You will need an amniocentesis procedure if you're over 35, which carries a risk (albeit small) of miscarriage. Can you handle all of these statistics? Can you handle the risk of Down's syndrome if you opt not to have an amniocentesis?

5. How much technological intervention is involved with each conception? If you're conceiving spontaneously with no fertility drugs and no ART procedures, obviously each conception attempt will involve less financial and emotional strain. You'll also need to take the above guidelines into consideration.

6. How has the loss affected your relationship with your partner? If the stress of your pregnancy loss or losses is straining your relationship, can it survive another loss? Or even the *risk* of a loss?

7. How are you? Are you a basket case at work? Are you having repeated nightmares? Are you sleeping? Are you depressed? Are you consumed with the loss/losses? Are you still in mourning? You shouldn't try again unless you're in good, emotional health, which leads us to the next guideline.

8. Have you sought out counseling of some kind? No one is emotionally "fine" after even a single episode of pregnancy loss. You need to seek out other couples who've gone through the experience and to air your feelings to a knowlegeable, qualified counselor. Again, you shouldn't attempt another pregnancy unless you're both in solid emotional shape.

Some of you may take the above guidelines, as well as those provided in chapter 8, move on to the final chapter, "All the Alternatives." Some of you may have stopped reading this book long ago and are into your second or third trimester of a normal pregnancy (a fate I wish for all of you). Nevertheless, for many couples dealing with unsalvageable fertility problems (see also chapters 4, 5, and 6), the next chapter is one not to miss. Alternatives mean *options*, not failure.

10

All the Alternatives

Throughout this book, each of you will have radically different fertility journeys, and different outcomes to those journeys. Some of you may have solved your fertility barrier by simply adjusting your lifestyle habits. Some of you may have found a specific problem that was easily remedied through medical treatment. Some of you may have required more aggressive treatments involving fertility drugs or surgery, while some of you may have opted for one of the many assisted reproductive technology (ART) methods. Some of you may have conceived but have experienced one or more episodes of pregnancy loss. And, hopefully, many of you are well on your way to successful pregnancies.

Yet happy endings to infertility are usually not that simple. Somewhere along the way, when biological conception isn't happening, many of your different journeys will converge on one word: *alternatives*. Yes, there are alternate, fulfilling lifestyle choices that do not involve biological parenting. This chapter will discuss all the alternatives you can consider, but since many of the topics covered here can become books in themselves, please look on this chapter as an introduction to alternatives, not as a detailed treatise on the subject.

In addition to covering topics such as adoption, social parenting, and childfree living, there are some issues you need to deal with first: refusal of treatment and stopping treatment. These are decisions you need to make *before* you consider other options to parenting. Unfortunately, you won't find a peaceful end to your struggle until you face these very tough choices.

Refusal of Treatment

Although many people look upon infertility as an "illness" that requires treatment, there are few causes of infertility that are life-threatening. In other words, many conditions that cause infertility are compatible with a full life expectancy. Obviously, conditions such as cancer, infections, or abcesses would need immediate attention. But many hormonal imbalances, genetic or anatomical anomalies, or diseases such as mild endometriosis do not technically require treatment. Limited time and financial resources are very real considerations when you contemplate treatment. For some, treatments can take place only with great financial sacrifice: second mortgages, bank loans, loans from family members or friends, sales of cars and personal possessions, lost income from time off work. Sometimes, lost *jobs* due to poor performance or *too* much time off can be the consequence of treatment.

Refusal of treatment also has a social stigma attached to it. Other couples— both fertile and infertile—may view your decision as selfish and say things like, "You obviously don't want a child badly enough to make the *necessary* sacrifices." Parents may view your decision as a personal affront to deny them grandchildren. Refusal of treatment is a highly individual choice. There is no right or wrong candidate for this decision. I've provided guidelines that will help you decipher whether this very personal choice is a valid decision for *you*. This list was compiled through a variety of sources, including couples who have chosen not to seek treatment.

Guidelines for Making Your Choice

1. *Have you had a workup?* I suspect many of you reading this chapter haven't even *seen* a doctor yet! At least find out what the cause of your infertility is before you decide to "refuse." What if you have chlamydia or prostatitis? These infections could lead to other health problems that antibiotics can avert.

2. *Is your problem easily treated?* There's a big difference between taking antibiotics for an infection and having reconstructive surgery. Does your treatment involve a few urine samples (for retrograde ejaculation) or undergoing a vasovasostomy? Does the treatment involve some lifestyle adjustments or fertility drugs? In other words, is treatment invasive or noninvasive? Time-consuming or incredibly involved? Refusing a simple treatment may lead to regrets down the road.

3. *Is the treatment expensive?* Everyone has a different definition of "expensive," but if the cost of your treatment will interfere with your mortgage payments and other essential bills, you probably can't afford it without financial aid. (Don't be coerced by friends who may taunt you with: "It's *just* another thousand a month? We spend that on eating out alone!" Or comments like: "That's *nothing* for what you're getting in return!")

4. *What financial aid is available?* Have you looked into this? If you're in good financial shape

(i.e., a low-risk borrower from a bank's perspective), a low-interest loan or refinancing a previous loan or mortgage may make your treatment affordable. On the other hand, if you're already in debt up to your eyeballs, the stress of treatment and paying for it might break you. Finally, if you have a poor credit history and no bank will give you a loan, this will also factor into your decision.

5. *What are the health risks of your treatment?* Chapter 7 describes all the risks involved with some fertility drugs, which may be enough to turn off any woman. Some people have se- vere reactions to anesthetics; others have chronic conditions that may cause adverse re- action to recommended treatments. If you don't want to risk future or short-term health problems from various drugs, this is a valid reason for not going ahead.

6. *What are your spiritual beliefs?* Some people truly feel that if they are meant to have chil- dren, it will happen naturally. This is absolutely valid.

7. *What are your moral beliefs?* Do you have a problem with the "playing God" overtones in- volved with fertility drugs and many ART procedures? If you do, this is a perfectly valid reason to refuse treatment.

8. *How does your partner feel about treatment?* This is a decision you need to make *together*. Some of the factors you'll need to look at: Who has the problem. Whose body will re- quire treatment and/or drugs? If you can't agree, you'll need to sort this out before you come to a final decision about treatment. Sometimes compromising and trying a *single* cycle of treatment (as opposed to the usual three to six months) solves the dilemma.

Stopping Treatment

The issue of stopping treatment is a concern for couples who are taking fertility drugs alone or in combination with an ART procedure. These treatments can become addictive unless you define when "enough is enough" *before* you start. Many couples report that the addiction lies in the hopefulness at the beginning of each new cycle. However, as each menstrual flow arrives, the de- spair gets deeper and deeper until you can't dig yourself out. Treatment is like being addicted to a miracle. "Just one more cycle and then we'll stop" can go on for longer than the recommended cycle-length of the fertiity drugs, and in some cases, for longer than two years, an eternity for fer- tility treatments.

Before you begin your treatment, you should have set down your own *financial* limits and *time* limits. For example, some couples plan for three in vitro fertilization (IVF) cycles and one gamete intrafallopian transfer (GIFT) cycle. Some couples plan for three clomiphene citrate cycles and one IVF cycle. You should then discuss a fallback plan in case treatments don't work. This may include adoption, childfree living, or plans to continue to try to conceive naturally (as may be the case for unexplained infertility, irregular cycles, or borderline low sperm count).

One couple with unexplained infertility actually went on oral contraception after their treatment cycle because the hopefulness/despair merry-go-round at the beginning of each natural cycle, and the beginning of each *period*, was just too much for them to handle emotionally. For this couple, oral contraception was the only way they could get on with their lives.

The Issue of Failure

For some, stopping treatment is admitting defeat or failure. Yet in the general fertile population, few will sacrifice what *you* have to reproduce. Issues like child abuse, deadbeat parents, and unwanted children infuriate those of us who cannot conceive. Where's the fairness in denying so many committed parents-to-be of biological reproduction when, clearly, so many people who *don't* deserve to be parents can reproduce at the drop of a hat? There is no fairness.

For philosophers, the "problem of evil" is what has kept the question of deity in a fiery debate over the centuries (i.e., "If there is a God, why is there so much evil in the world?"). For infertile couples, the justice in who gets to reproduce and who doesn't is a philosophical and spiritual quandary. For many, it is the spiritual straw that may turn us away from religion, or draw us into it.

STOP Signs

For every person in treatment, there are different STOP signs that tell him or her that "enough is enough." The following is a list of signs compiled from other couples' experiences. If you're currently in treatment and you've seen one of the emotional and/or physical signs below, it may be time for *you* to stop.

1. The fertility drugs are causing painful or adverse symptoms, ranging from physical pain to severe mood swings.
2. You're already in debt and cannot afford another cycle.
3. You cannot stand to be around anyone but your partner and your doctor. You can't remember the last time you chatted with a friend.

4. You can't remember the last time you did anything for pleasure—reading, sports, going to a movie—that did *not* revolve around infertility.
5. You and/or your partner are incapable of becoming sexually aroused just for "fun."
6. You eat, drink, and sleep infertility. You're so obsessed about your infertility that it's interfering with your job, your sex life, your social network, and your relationship with your partner.
7. You're showing signs of depression: apathy, loss of interest in formerly pleasurable activities, change in appetite (usually decreased), fatigue, guilt, self-loathing, suicidal thoughts, poor concentration and memory, sleeplessness (waking early and not going back to sleep), and anxiety.

Parenting Without Pregnancy

You can still parent a child without experiencing pregnancy and childbirth. In fact, this is often a satisfying solution to many infertile couples and is preferable to assisted reproduction procedures. Even in a book devoted to infertility issues, it's not possible to cover the range of adoption scenarios that exist, or the range of issues that surround each individual scenario, be it open, private/independent arrangements, or international adoptions. Entire books have been written about just one of the arrangements discussed in this chapter. Therefore, consider this a "get started" section about adoption, and consult the appendix for adoption resources. They can direct you to more detailed books that devote adequate space to the subject.

Creating Spiritual Offspring: Adoption

Adopting after the experience of infertility means that you need to revise your original definitions of parenting. There is considerable stress involved with repeated workups and reversing certain causes of infertility. Many couples will and *should* ask, "Is all this worth it for a biological child?" After reviewing their true motivations for wanting a biological child, many couples will *not* pursue infertility testing and assisted conception, and decide to love a child that's already here. This is a logical decision, considering how many unwanted children there are who *need* parents! Unfortunately, there are two societal myths that interfere with a couple's decision to adopt: "Biological parents make *better* parents, and biological children make *better* children. *This just isn't true!*

I liken the decision to adopt to the experience of finding a lifetime partner. When we're in our teens, most of us fantasize about an ideal mate. The fantasy mate is far removed, of course, from *realistic* human relationships. Yet these fantasies are perfectly normal; *everyone* does it! After a while we learn through our own individual processes, to let go of our fantasy mate. It is usually around this time that we meet our lifetime partner, who might have been there all along, or who we may seem to suddenly meet (when in fact it's more a case of recognizing qualities you were previously blind to). And, in cases where we *do* meet who we *think* is our fantasy mate, there is a period of "let down" when that person makes a mistake and we are forced to admit that he of she really *isn't* perfect after all. Ultimately, whether we've met that person on a blind date, through the personals, or because we spilled coffee on him or her, most of us feel as though that person is supposed to be in our lives. If we didn't, we wouldn't make a lifelong commitment.

The process of adopting a child is similar. For all couples, there is a "fantasy child" that doesn't reflect the realistic experience of being a parent at all. Parents who have biological children soon discover that there is far less fantasy involved than hard reality when it comes to the real McCoy. But for an infertile couple, that fantasy child becomes a stronger image, which only reinforces the pain of infertility. The real truth is, having a biological child is *no* guarantee of lifelong happiness! To emphasize this point, an award-winning foreign TV commercial went to hilarious extents. The commercial opens with the line: "Two good reasons to use Brand X Condoms." Then, we are shown two sets of proud parents, circa 1900, fawning over their newborns. Their names flash across the screen: "Mr. and Mrs. Hitler" and "Mr. and Mrs. Mussolini."

The point is that couples who choose adoption need to let go of their "fantasy" child and accept that the child they're supposed to be with is not biological offspring, but *spiritual* offspring.

A Brief History of Adoption

Until the 1970s, adoptions in North America were handled by public or private agencies that had more babies up for adoption than couples willing to parent them. Yet because of greater sophistication regarding birth control, the legalization of abortion, and the destigmatization of parenting a child outside of marriage, there are more couples seeking to adopt a baby, than there are available babies. In the 1980s and early 1990s, more than half of *all* North American adoptions were *independent adoptions* (a.k.a. *private adoption*). This is when birth parents are actively involved in finding an adoptive family. Although public and private agency adoption is still alive and well, the process usually takes longer and many of these agencies still allow no contact between the birth parents and adoptive parents.

It's crucial to note, though, that if you're willing to adopt an older child, a child who is a visible minority (even if you are, too), or a special needs child, you can expect a child from a public or private agency almost immediately. The average wait in these same agencies for a Caucasian infant is *four to eight years*. The wait is much less through independent/private adoption, translating into roughly six to nine months.

Today, many couples need to go outside of their countries to adopt an infant or toddler, which is known as international adoption. I'll discuss some of the issues you need to be aware of if you're going the international route.

Getting Started

The maze of decisions, bureaucracy, and paperwork can be extremely overwhelming once you make your decision to adopt. The following are guidelines I've compiled from a number of sources to help you take your own baby steps into the adoption process.

General steps

1. *Contact local adoption and infertility support groups*. Your best source of information regarding adopting are from people who live in your community who have gone through the process successfully. Pick as many brains as you can. Infertility groups are also tremendous sources of information. Many people who join these support groups already have one or more adopted children.
2. *Search for government programs*. Whether these programs are at the local/municipal, state/provincial, or the federal level, find out *what* programs exist that can help you adopt a child in your own country or internationally.
3. *Read everything you can on the subject*. Before you decide what kind of adoption process is right for you, educate yourself about what's involved with each route: costs, time/wait, available children, necessary paperwork, and so on.
4. *Lawyer-shop*. Don't hire anyone yet. Just shop around and ask people you know and trust. (Use some of the strategies outlined in chapter 1.) Ask people you've met through the support group venue. To avoid the average $350 consultation fee, ask if the lawyer can send you information on his or her practice or give you names of satisfied clients. Ask if you can take the lawyer out to lunch for an hour or so just to meet. (Once you discuss your case, the lawyer may charge you.) Or, as a last resort, ask for a 10-minute meeting.

This will give you a chance to check out the office, the feel, the lawyer's initial persona, and so on.

5. *Beware of adoption "facilitator" services.* These usually translate into high fees with few leads.

6. *Hire a lawyer who specializes in adoption.* Do this before you tell anyone about your decision to adopt. That way, if you get an immediate lead, you'll have your lawyer there to negotiate the details. (If you're going the international route, see the separate section below.)

7. *Tell everyone and his or her dog that you want to adopt.* Even if you're planning on adopting internationally, the more people who know about your situation, the more likely you are of finding a child.

Independent Adoption (a.k.a. Private Adoption)

In independent adoption, the adoptive parents take an active role in searching for an infant to adopt. A lawyer represents the adoptive parents and makes all the legal arrangements for the adoption. The birth parents consent to placing the child directly with the adoptive parents, rather than using an agency as the middleperson. Usually, the birth mother is found during the later stages of pregnancy, and the baby goes directly from the hospital into the adoptive parents' home.

There are no set rules to adopting independently, but the best method is to find a family law practitioner who specializes in adoption. First, lawyers who specialize in adoption have a network of contacts that may lead to a child sooner. Second, it's crucial to have someone who can expertly negotiate a clear, contractual arrangement with the birth parents to avoid future legal battles over the child. Make sure that you and your lawyer sign a contract or agreement that clearly states costs in various scenarios, and outlines fees under more complex circumstances (such as adopting twins or siblings, waiting longer than expected, and so on). Your lawyer should also make sure that any money that's exchanged between you and the birth parents is confidential (i.e., disbursing all money through an escrow account).

Announce your decision to everyone you can think of. Ask people to put feelers out for available children, and you may just get the call you've been waiting for: "The woman my aunt's cousin's sister works with is pregnant and unmarried and looking for a home for her child."

The next step is conducting a campaign, just as you would if you were starting a small business. Set up an unlisted 1-800 number. Then create a print advertisement to be placed in various newspapers and specialty magazines. The headline may go something like: "30-something

Couple Looking to Adopt." The body copy may read something like: "We're very eager to share our love with a child and form a family. Sadly, we cannot have children of our own, but we want to offer our love, values, and sense of family to a child who needs a home. For more information, call us at 1-800-555-5555." You may also want to consider a radio ad and even a television ad (on cheaper, cable-access stations) if your media budget permits. Some couples have even gone as far as using billboards to advertise their message.

Then, you'll need to conduct a *direct-mail* campaign. Compile the names and addresses of obstetricians, hospitals, clergy, family doctors, other family law practitioners, abortion counselors, high school counselors, student health services, women's health clinics, and other adoption services. (There are companies that have mailing lists you can purchase.) A good number to work with is about 1,000. Then, write one common, one- to two-page letter to these people stating who you are, why you want to adopt, where you live, what your income is, what your cultural/religious beliefs are, what your professions are, and how you can be contacted at all times (business and home numbers, and numbers of friends or family in case you're away). You should also include your 1-800 number and a business card. Photos of yourselves (one picture with two of you in an embrace), your home, other family members, and pets are also helpful. Attach letters of recommendation from colleagues or friends, as well as your professional resumes, so your work experience and education are crystal clear. Send out this package and see if you get a response.

Once you find your lead, you and your lawyer will work out financial details that may involve paying for the birth mother's medical and counseling expenses, some living expenses that pertain to the health of the child while the birth mother is pregnant, and, of course, all prenatal and neonatal medical expenses. You should not be expected to pay enormous sums of money for the child (a fee of, say, $20,000, over and above all reasonable expenses). Keep in mind that some sort of fee to the birth mother may be expected as a way of compensation, but this usually isn't done. (Compensation fees for the birth mother are legal in some places and illegal in others.)

There are agencies that claim to be independent adoption facilitators, but there are numerous horror stories about many of these services, which require an up-front nonrefundable fee and eventually yield no leads. Be careful. Ask to see a list of satisfied clients and check out the credentials of the people running the agency first.

If all goes well and you've found a birth mother who consents to place her child with you, you'll need to cough up your birth certificates, marriage certificates, medical records, notarized current financial statements, income tax returns, and employer letters verifying your position and salary. You'll also need to have what's known as a "home study" done. This is where a social worker (either independent, or as part of an agency) comes into your home and asks you invasive questions about your private life, assesses your home and neighborhood, assesses your personal qualities and values, and so on. A report is prepared for the birth parents prior to their consent. This same social worker may conduct follow-up visits during the first six months you have the child.

Again, independent/private adoptions are the most popular form of adoption in North America. (Often, many couples will move on to international adoption if they're unsuccessful in adopting independently.)

The independent steps

The following is a summary of the general steps involved with independent/private adoptions:

1. Self-educate (read, network with other adoptive parents, and so on).
2. Hire your lawyer. (See above for more details.)
3. Assemble your paperwork (birth/marriage certificates, letters of recommendation.)
4. Contact a certified social worker to do your home study. (This may also be a later step once you find the birth parents.)
5. Install an unlisted 800 number and plan your ad and direct-mail campaign.

Steps when you get a response...

1. Put together a list of interested birth parents and screen out the "undesirables" (you'll have your own criteria for this)
2. Make a short list of birth parent candidates and ask to meet them *with your lawyer present*. Keep in mind that it's a birth parent's market, though. They may not want to do this and wish to meet with you privately without disclosing any identifying information, or they may not want to meet until the child is transferred to you.
3. Have your lawyer do all the necessary checking regarding background, medical records, test results for HIV, alcohol, or drugs. Your lawyer will also help the birth parents find legal representation.
4. Contact your pediatrician and let him or her know that information about the child might be forwarded in the near future.
5. Wait for the birth of the child.

Open or shut?

Independent adoptions may be open, semi-open, or closed. In an open adoption, you meet the birth parents in person and share full identifying information. You may also hve ongoing contact over the years, either in person or through correspondence. The birth parents may visit the child as frequently as you and they are comfortable with, and may even become extended family members. This is a new and healthy approach to adoption, but it only works if *all* parties involved are mature individuals.

In a semi-open adoption, you meet the birth parents but they don't give you any identifying information about themselves. In turn, you agree to send them pictures and updates on the child for a limited period of time, to be negotiated by your lawyer.

In a closed adoption, you never meet the birth parents and have everything done through your lawyer. You essentially have no direct contact with the birth parents and you don't send them any pictures or updates on the child.

Public and Private Agencies

Private adoption shouldn't be confused with private *agency* adoption. There's a huge difference. Official adoption agencies are state- or provincially regulated private or public agencies that "project manage" the adoption from beginning to end. While the wait can be longer, these adoptions are considered safer in that there's less risk of the birth parents changing their minds; the birth parents have relinquished their legal rights to the children, placing them in the agency's care. However, as long as you have a lawyer handling your independent adoption, this perception of more safety is a bit of a myth.

The usual process involves contacting the agency, being informally screened, and discussing the agency's fees and rules. The agency will then screen you for acceptability before they put you on a waiting list. They'll also conduct a home study (in fact, the home studies now required for independent adoptions were borrowed from these agencies). Then the wait begins. When a child is placed with you, there is a 3–12 month adjustment period you'll have to live through until the child is legally yours. If there are adjustment problems, a social worker will try to resolve the problem rather than taking away the child.

The only steps involved in this process are educating yourself about the types of adoptions possible *before* choosing this one, and then shopping around for the agency you think will best serve you. Try to use an agency that someone has referred to you. You should also have a lawyer representing you who can negotiate any documents or contracts you need to sign, and find anything potentially fishy about a contract you sign.

International Adoption

If you're willing to spring for airfare and a long list of other costs, you might consider this option. Outside of North America, there is a very high orphan population. You'll need an immigration lawyer and possibly a family law practitioner to help you, but the exact process involved in an independent adoption really depends on the *country* you want to adopt from. Every country has its own rules and required documentation. Throughout North America, there are consultant agencies set up to act as a liaison between your own country and the child's country. *You cannot get anywhere without a liaison.* These liaisons locate foreign child-placing sources on your behalf. They'll make contact with the foreign source and will assist you in compiling your documents.

International adoption is a huge topic that I cannot possibly do justice to in one section. However, I've outlined some of the requirements involved for the most popular regions. For all regions, it's important that the adoptive parents try to visit the country prior to adopting. In many cases, one parent can visit the country and bring the child back to North America within a couple of weeks. There are lists of international adoption agencies and liaison services through local adoption networks, infertility networks, and departments of immigration.

Europe

Any married couple of any age, regardless of divorce history or number of previous children, may adopt here. Europe is also open to single parents. Each country in Europe monitors adoption through local courts of the country of the adoptive parents and of the child. These children are of Byelorussian, Ukrainian, Russian, Slovakian, and other European origin. Most of these children are either in orphanages or hospitals, where they were abandoned by their unmarried mothers at birth. There is often no reliable information about their histories. Many of the children are malnourished and therefore have slightly stunted physical growth that resumes normally once they're fed and clothed properly. There are many babies that are newborn or older that are immediately available.

Immigration requirements for the United States and Canada involve filing various documents and fees with local and federal immigration services so that your child can receive a visa to travel back to North America. The entire process, including application fees, registration fees, and dossier fees, can cost roughly $10,000 or more. This does not include transportation costs or legal fees. The entire process costs $40,000 (a conservative estimate).

China

Married couples 35 years or older without children may adopt, while single adults are not given priority. If you're younger than 35 or already have children, some exceptions may be made, but don't count on it. Look for another country. You must be willing to adopt girls, because generally the only children available are girls ranging from newborn to two years old. Infants from Hunan and Jiangsu provinces are available, and some will have correctable handicaps. You're looking at roughly the same costs as a European adoption, once you factor in legal fees and plane fares.

Latin America (Central and South America and Mexico)

Couples over 25 years of age who are childless will be given preference to couples who already have one or more children. The countries most popular include Bolivia, Brazil, Chile, Colombia, Ecuador, Guatemala, Honduras, Panama, and Peru. Paraguay and Mexico are also popular areas. The children are mostly of Hispanic or Indian heritage and, in one or two countries, children of African heritage are available. The costs involved are roughly the same as a European adoption.

Documentation requirements

1. Certified birth certificates for each adoptive parent and family member
2. Certified marriage license and/or divorce decrees
3. Financial statement
4. Medical examination for each adoptive parent and each family member
5. Police clearance forms by local police, stating that each adoptive parent has no criminal record
6. Advanced approval through either the Immigration and Naturalization Service (advance processing approval document I 171-H) in the United States, or Immigration Canada (Undertaking of Assistance document, issued by Immigration Canada and accompanied by the Letter of No-Involvement, issued by MCSS Adoption Desk for immigration purposes)
7. Approved home study by licensed agency
8. Employment letter for each adoptive parent
9. Letters of reference
10. Photo of home and adoptive parents
11. Intention to adopt form (prepared by your liaison agency)
12. Power of attorney (prepared by your liaison agency)
13. Passport
14. Photocopy of your most recent tax form

Two sets of your documents need to be supplied: one set in English, for North American proceedings, and one set in the language of the country you're adopting from, for the adoption proceedings in that country

Adoption Myths

"So and so adopted and then got pregnant. If you start the process, you'll probably get pregnant, too!" This is one of those stories *every* infertile couple hears from a reliable source, who *swears* it really happened. Well, it *rarely* happens, and unfortunately, it's the kind of myth that's really not helpful for anyone looking to adopt. All you can do is reply with something like, "If I wanted to get pregnant, I'd (still) be in treatment."

Myth number two: "Well, you *know*, these kids might have learning disabilities and other problems . . ." *This is the exception, not the rule.* Although it's true that many older children who are put up for adoption may have been born to drug-abusing mothers or raised for a time in an abusive home, no agency in the 1990s will withhold this information from you. A child's medical records and history will be *made absolutely clear to you!* If the child you want to adopt is dysfunctional emotionally, this will surface during your adjustment period, before the adoption is legal. The child may take longer to trust you or may need extra therapy, but these problems are usually workable. In more extreme cases, the agency will categorize that child as a "special needs" child from the outset, so any emotional problems will come as no surprise, and you'll *choose* whether you want to take them on.

In an international adoption, children's medical histories are less straightforward. You can have the child checked out by a qualified pediatrician before you agree to take him or her back to North America. If you suspect an abusive background, appropriate therapy and your influence as a loving parent can help that child overcome it.

However, more adoptions now go the independent route anyway, which means that you'll meet the birth parents (or at least the birth mother) and will have complete access to the parents' and child's medical histories. These stipulations can be negotiated in your contract!

As for the learning disability issue and psychological adjustment problems, this is a societal bias. All children, whether biological or adopted, may experience periods of emotional turmoil. It's all part of the precarious nature of life on earth. This can be caused by an unstable home environment, by an experience that traumatizes the child (witnessing something frightening, getting lost, etc.), or by external factors, such as school adjustment problems. How well your child adjusts to life in general has more to do with who *you* are as a parent. If you're a psychologically stable, loving, and mature person, this will have an impact on how well your child adjusts to the emotional challenges (including finding out about the adoption) he or she will confront. Remember, *nobody* is immune to trauma and adversity.

Childfree Living

Every family has that one kindly aunt and uncle who "never had any children." And, until you *yourself* have struggled with infertility, you probably never wondered *why* they had no children; you just accepted it. Well, if that aunt and uncle of yours are now seniors, in *their* day they could have adopted from a wide assortment of newborns (of which there is now a shortage for white, middle-class infertile couples). *But they didn't.* Today, they probably live comfortably in a small condo somewhere, travel a great deal, are enjoying their retirement, and dote on a large selection of nieces and nephews. When they pass on, they'll probably leave their money to their "favorite" niece or nephew and will always be fondly remembered.

Now, compare *that* lifestyle to the "other" aunt and uncle who have three miserable sons who "eat their hearts out." Everyone in the family knows that these sons scammed their own parents out of their life savings. One son is a stingy businessman who nobody in the family likes, the other is a cocaine addict who sold his father's collector's edition car to buy more coke, while the third son is a bum and has never worked an honest day in his life!

I exaggerate these two lifestyles to point out that there is no guarantee of happiness either way. Some couples with children wish they'd never had them; couples with no children may regret it. The decision *itself* is not as important as how *comfortable you are with your choice.*

In the past, a childfree lifestyle was often a *political* decision for many couples. During the 1950s and 1960s, many couples chose this because they feared a nuclear holocaust. By the 1970s, the issue of overpopulation became the motivating factor for the choice. Yet by the 1980s, childfree living became a symbol of infertility and failure, a symbol that has prevailed into the 1990s. This is a pity, considering what a liberating lifestyle option it can be. Obviously, you'll need to review your original reasons for wanting children before you make this choice. You'll also need to research the decision: interview other couples who are living childfree and investigate *their* lifestyle. Interview couples with children and find out how much of their own lives are sacrificed.

Some fertile couples are choosing childfree living because of environmental and financial concerns. Many truly feel the world is an environmental disaster area and do not wish to raise children in a world of questionable health hazards. Other couples find that they can barely meet their bills as it is, and opt not to add more stress to an already badly strained budget. Remember, parenting is a selfless, largely self-sacrificing job. Choosing a childfree lifestyle may be an appealing option in an economically turbulent and difficult world.

Some of the traditional reasons for having children were *purely* economic. Children, many people thought, guaranteed financial security in old age. Today, with so many college-educated adults living at home because they cannot get jobs, the economic benefits of progeny are no longer visible. And you'll find that most senior-age parents of financially successful children today do not want to be a financial burden and will choose to be independent as long as they can. Another traditional reason for having children was fear of loneliness in one's old age. Twenty years from now, the majority of the population will be over age 65. You won't be lonely.

The Benefit Package

1. *Freedom.* You may have the time and extra money down the road for all the things you dreamed of: going back to school for that second degree, buying a vacation home, traveling, early retirement, or whatever you want.
2. *Control of your life.* When you have children, you lose a certain amount of control over your own life. Children can have lots of problems. They may have difficulty at school; they get sick; they have accidents; they get in trouble; they get *pregnant*; and so on. You never stop being a parent.
3. *Self-expansion.* You'll have the time to explore parts of yourself that you never knew existed, because you'll have time to *yourself*. Insights about your life, your gifts, your talents, your desires, your interests can be explored. Here are two images to keep in mind: Katharine Hepburn at age 70, and any other 70-year-old whose life was ruined because of his or her children. I'll take Katharine Hepburn's life any day.

At any rate, whatever your reasons are for living childfree, the decision is, of course, *reversible* anytime you wish.

Social Parenting

This is what you get when you cross adoption with childfree living. You can become involved with the children in your life: nieces, nephews, godchildren, or friends' children. One woman I interviewed has a toy chest and children's book library that is the envy of all her friends. She spends precious quality time with many of her friends' children of all ages. The children love her, the parents love it because they get a break from their kids, and she benefits enormously. She has become that one special grown-up the children can confide in, yet she can also influence their developing values and skills. She shares in their successes and trials of childhood. "I've never met a child who doesn't have room to love one more person," she tells me.

The Last Word

If you're like me, this may be the first section you've turned to in this book. Whether you're just entering the planning stages of conception and have no idea whether you're fertile or not, are going through a conception struggle or workup, have been experiencing repeated miscarriages, are undergoing treatment, or are experiencing secondary infertility, you haven't been left out of this fertility book. You'll find many of the answers to your questions here, as well as information regarding several difficult issues that may be concerning you. You'll learn how lifestyle or work habits affect your fertility, how to find a fertility specialist, how to gauge your menstrual cycle, the many causes of and treatments for infertility, and all the alternatives to biological parenting. Take this book to the doctor with you, read it, and share it with your friends. Good luck and good health.

Bibliography

Chapter 1

Cain, Joanna M., M.D., and Albert R. Jonsen. "Specialists and Generalists in Obstetrics and Gynecology: Conflicts of Interest in Referral and an Ethical Alternative." *The Jacobs Institute of Women's Health* 2, no. 3 (Fall 1992).

Chez, Ronald A., M.D., and Franklin J. Apfel, M.D. "Women's Health Care: Rights and Responsibilities." *The Jacobs Institute of Women's Health* 2, no. 3 (Fall 1992).

Dewitt, Don, M.D. "Family Physicians, Pap Smears, and Colposcopy." *American Family Physician*, January 1992.

Infertility: Your Role on the Medical Team. Utica, N.Y.: Ferre Institute, Inc., 1994.

Maleskey, Gale and Charles B. Inlander. "Book Extra: What You Should Know About Pap Tests." *People's Medical Society Newsletter* 10 (April 1991).

———. *Take This Book to the Gynecologist with You: A Consumer's Guide to Women's Health*. New York: Addison-Wesley, 1991.

Maurer, Janet, M.D. *How to Talk to Your Doctor*. New York: Simon & Schuster, 1986.

Morales, Karla, and Charles B. Inlander. *Take This Book to the Obstetrician with You*. New York: Addison-Wesley, 1991.

"Patient's Bill of Rights." Ottawa: Infertility Awareness Association of Canada patient information,1994.

Rees, Susan. "Doubting Our Doctors," *Weight Watchers*, May 1993.

Rosenthal, M. Sara. *The Gynecological Sourcebook*, Los Angeles: Lowell House, 1994.

———. *The Pregnancy Sourcebook*. Los Angeles: Lowell House, 1994.

———. *The Thyroid Sourcebook*. Los Angeles: Lowell House, 1993.

Chapter 2

Miller Chenier, Nancy. *Reproductive Hazards at Work: Men, Women, and the Fertility Gamble*. Ottawa: Canadian Advisory Council on the Status of Women, 1982.

Petrenko, Alexa. "Creating Fertile Ground: Safe and Natural Approaches to Overcoming Infertility." *Vitality*, November 1992.

Rowland, Andrew S., Donna Day Baird, Clarice R. Weinberg, David L. Shore, Carl M. Shy, M.D., and Allen J.Wilcox, M.D. "Reduced Fertility Among Women Employed as Dental Assistants Exposed to High Levels of Nitrous Oxide." *New England Journal of Medicine*, October 1, 1992.

"Sperm-density Study Surprising." *Globe and Mail*, 10 June 1994.

Chapter 3

"Basal Body Temperature Charts." Mississauga, Ontario: Serono Canada, Inc. patient information, 1994.

Garner, Catherine H., and Grant W. Patton, M.D. *Pathways to Parenthood*. Mississauga, Ontario: Serono Canada, Inc., 1994.

"Getting Pregnant, Naturally." Toronto: Justisse Group client information, 1994.

"Getting Pregnant Naturally Depends on Your Combined Fertility." Toronto: Justisse Group client information, 1994.

"Justisse Method for Fertility Management." Toronto: Justisse Group client information, 1994.

Rosenthal, M. Sara. *The Gynecological Sourcebook*. Los Angeles: Lowell House, 1994.

"Temperature Record." Ottawa: Infertility Awareness Association of Canada client information, 1994.

Chapter 4

Adler, Alexis. "The Importance of Semen Analysis in Assessing Male Factor Infertility." Ottawa: Infertility Awareness Association of Canada client information, 1994.

Blank, William, M.D. "Electroejaculation and Vibratory Stimulation for Sperm Retrieval in Men With Ejaculatory Disturbances." Ottawa: Infertility Awareness Association of Canada client information, 1994.

Braverman, Andrea Mechanick. "The Psychosocial Issues in Male Infertility." Ottawa: Infertility Awareness Association of Canada client information, 1994.

"Getting Pregnant Naturally Depends on Your Combined Fertility." Toronto: Justisse Group client information, 1994.

Greendale, Gail, et al. "The Relationship of Chlamydia Trachomatis Infection and Male Infertility." *The American Journal of Public Health*, July 1993.

"Increase of Cyclophosphamide on Long-term Reduction in Sperm Count in Men Treated with Combination Chemotherapy for Ewing and Soft-tissue Sarcomas," by M.L. Meistrich, et al. *Cancer Weekly*, December 14, 1992.

The Infertility Workup: What to Expect. Utica NY: Ferre Institute, Inc.

Jackson, Ted. "Male Infertility: Breaking the Silence." Ottawa: The Infertility Awareness Association of Canada client information, 1994.

Jarvi, Keith, M.D. Interview with author. Mt. Sinai Hospital, Toronto, Ontario, 1994.

Karpen, Maxine. "Varicocele Linked to Ongoing Decline in Fertility." Ottawa: Infertility Awareness Association of Canada client informtion, 1994.

Lipshultz, M.D. *Male Infertility*. Serono Symposia, USA, 1993.

Myers, Michael, M.D. "Male Gender-related Issues in Reproductive Technology." *Psychiatric Aspects of Reproductive Technology*. Washington, D.C.: American Psychiatric Press, 1990.

Shlagman, Roy. "Infertility: A Male Perspective." Somerville, MA: Resolve client information, 1994.

Zoldbrod, Aline P. "Decisionmaking in Male Infertility." Patient information handout, November 1987.

———. "Men's Reaction to Infertility: Their Feelings are Concealed." *Insights Into Infertility* newsletter,Summer 1991. Distributed by Infertility Awareness Association of Canada.

Chapter 5

Batista, Marcelo, et al. "Comparative Analysis of Progesterone and Placental Protein Measurements in the Evaluation of Luteal Function."*American Journal of Obstetrics and Gynecology*, May 1993.

Doherty, Carolyn M., Bruce Silver, Zvi Binor, Mary Wood Molo, and Ewa Radwanska. "Transvaginal Ultrasonography and the Assessment of Luteal Phase Endometrium." *American Journal of Obstetrics and Gynecology*, June 1993.

Domar, Alice D., Alexis Broome, Patricia Zuttermeister, Machelle Seibel, M.D., and Richard Friedman. "The Prevalence and Predictability of Depression in Infertile Women." *Fertility and Sterility* 58, no. 6, (December 1992).

Fritz, Mark, Ronald Holmes, and Edward Keenan. "Effect of Clomiphene Citrate Treatment on Endometrial Estrogen and Progesterone Receptor Induction in Women." *American Journal of Obstetrics and Gynecology*, July 1991.

"General Guideline for Treatment of Infertility." Ottawa: Infertility Awareness Association of Canada client information.

The Infertility Workup: What to Expect. Utica, N.Y.: Ferre Institute, Inc.

Miller, Kathleen D. "Hodgkin's Disease: Impact on Childbearing." *The Journal of Perinatal and Neonatal Nursing*, March 1994.

Polycystic Ovarian Disease: A Guide for Patients. Birmingham, Alabama: American Fertility Society, 1994.

Rosenthal, M. Sara. *The Gynecological Sourcebook*. Los Angeles: Lowell House, 1994.

The Turner's Syndrome Society. Concord, Ontario: Turner's Syndrome Society of Canada patient information, 1994.

Chapter 6

Braverman, Andrea Mechanick. "The Psychosocial Issues in Male Infertility." Ottawa: Infertility Awareness Association of Canada. Ottawa client information..

Gonzales, Frank, Denise Hatala, and Leon Speroff. "Adrenal and Ovarian Steroid Hormone Responses to Gonadotropin-releasing Hormone Agonist Treatment in Polycystic Ovary Syndrome." *American Journal of Obstetrics and Gynecology*, September 1991.

Jarvi, Keith, M.D. Interview with author. Mt. Sinai Hospital, Toronto, Ontario, 1994.

Lipshultz, M.D. *Male Infertility*. Norwell, MA: Serono Symposia, USA, 1993.

Polycystic Ovarian Disease: A Guide for Patients. Birmingham, Alabama: American Fertility Society patient information, 1994.

Rosenthal, M. Sara. *The Gynecological Sourcebook*. Los Angeles: Lowell House, 1994.

Shlagman, Roy. "Infertility: A Male Perspective." Somerville, MA.: Resolve client information, 1994.

Zoldbrod, Aline P. "Men's Reaction to Infertility: Their Feelings are Concealed." *Insights into Infertility* newsletter, Summer 1991.

Chapter 7

"Answers to Common Questions about Clomiphene Therapy." Mississauga, Ontario: Serono Canada Inc. patient information, 1994.

Baraldi, Rosanna. "Ovulation Inductors and DES: Is History Repeating Itself?" *DES Action* newsletter, published by DES Action USA, Spring 1991.

———. "Evaluation of Long-term Consequences of Drug Testing...Where is the Progress?" *DES Action* newsletter, published by DES Action USA, Summer 1992.

"Clomiphene Citrate Tablets." Jerusalem: Serono Laboratories, Inc.factsheet.

"Fertility Drugs May Raise Ovarian Cancer Risk." *Journal of the National Cancer Institute*, 85, no. 2 (January 20, 1993).

Fritz, Mark, Ronald Holmes, and Edward Keenan. "Effects of Clomiphene Citrate Treatment on Endometrial Estrogen and Progesterone Receptor Induction in Women." *American Journal of Obstetrics and Gynecology*, July, 1991.

Herman, Robin. "Dying to Conceive." *Mirabella*, July 1994.

Infertility Care with Humegon. Scarborough, Ontario: Organon Canada.

"Infertility Treatment Using Hormone-based Therapies Is Proven Safe and Effective." Serono, Corporate Communications North America news release.

Marrs, Richard, M.D. and Stuart Hartz. "Comments on the Possible Association Between Ovulation Inducing Agents and Ovarian Cancer." Birmingham Alabama: The American Fertility Society, January 1993.

"Menotropins (Systemic) Advice for the Patient." *Drug Information in Lay Language*, Edition 14 (1994).

"Metrodin." Aubonne, Switzerland: Serono Laboratories Inc.factsheet, 1994.

"No Proven Link Between Ovarian Cancer and Infertiltiy Drug Treatment." Serono, Corporate Communications North America news release, 1993.

"Ovarian Cancer Risk Assessed in Comprehensive Study." Stanford University Medical Center news release, January 13, 1993.

Ovulation Induction. Cambridge, England: Organon Laboratories, Ltd., 1994.

"Pergonal." Aubonne, Switzerland: Serono Laboratories Inc. factsheet.

Pergonal/Profasi Therapy. Mississauga, Ontario: Serono Canada.

Polycystic Ovarian Disease. Birmingham Alabama: American Fertility Society.

"Questions and Answers for the Metrodin Patient." Mississauga, Ontario: Serono Canada Inc. patient information.

"Risks of Ovarian Cancer." Mississauga, Ontario: Serono Canada Inc. factsheet.

Rosenthal, M. Sara. *The Gynecological Sourcebook.* Los Angeles: Lowell House, 1994.

Whittemore, Alice S, Robin Harris, Jacqueline Itnyre, and the Collaborative Ovarian Cancer Group. "Characteristics Relating to Ovarian Cancer Risk: Collaborative Analysis of 12 U.S. Case-Control Studies." *American Journal of Epidemiology* 136, no. 10 (1992).

Willemsen, Wim, Roy Kruitwagen, Bart Bastiaans, Ton Hanselaar, and Rune Rolland. "Ovarian Stimulation and Granulosa-Cell Tumor." *The Lancet*, April 17, 1993.

Chapter 8

Alikani, Mina, and Jacques Cohen. "Advances in Clinical Micromanipulation of Gametes and Embryos: Assisted Fertilization and Hatching." *Archives of Pathology and Laboratory Medicine* 116, no. 4 (April 1992).

ART: Assisted Reproductive Technologies. Mississauga, Ontario: Serona Canada, Inc.

Asch, Ricardo, H., M.D., and Serono Symposia, U.S.A. *GIFT: Gamete Intra-Fallopian Transfer.* Norwell, MA: Serono Symposia USA.

Assael, Shaun. "Immaculate Deception." *SmartMoney*, August 1993.

Charbonneau, Leo. "New Procedure Offers 'Truly Outstanding' Pregnancy Rates." Reprinted by Infertility Awareness Association, Canada, November, 1993.

Clayton, Christine E., and Gabor T. Kovacs. "AID Offspring: Initial Follow-up Study of 50 Couples." *The Medical Journal of Australia*, April 17, 1982.

Cohen, Jacques, Beth E. Talansky, Alexis Adler, Mina Alikani, and Zev Rosenwaks. "Controversies and Opinions in Clinical Microsurgical Fertilization." *Journal of Assisted Reproduction and Genetics* 9, no. 2 (1992).

Domar, Alice D., Patricia C. Zuttermeister, Machelle Seibel, M.D., and Herbert Benson, M.D. "Psychological Improvement in Infertile Women after Behavioral Treatment: A Replication." *Fertility and Sterility* 58, no. 1 (July, 1992).

———. "The Mind/Body Program for Infertility: A New Behavioral Treatment Apprach for Women with Infertility." *Fertility and Sterility* 53, no. 2 (February 1990).

"Donor Insemination: A New Beginning." Oakland, CA: The Sperm Bank of California patient information.

"Donor Sperm—A Happy Ending." *Lifeline* newsletter, LIFE Program, Toronto East General Hospital and IVF Canada, April 1993.

Gordon, Jon W. "Controversies in Assisted Reproduction: Current Unresolved Controversies in Micromanipulation-Assisted Fertilization." *Journal of Assisted Reproduction and Genetics* 9, no. 3 (June 1992).

"Guidelines for Oocyte Donation." *The American Fertility Society Supplement 1*: 59, no. 2 (February 1993).

"How To Choose an In Vitro Fertilization (IVF) Program." Ottawa: Infertility Awareness Association of Canada patient information.

Jones, Howard W. Jr., M.D., and James P. Toner, M.D. "Current Concepts: The Infertile Couple." *The New England Journal of Medicine*, December 1993.

Lasker, Judith N., and Susan Borg. *In Search of Parenthood: Coping with Infertility and High-Tech Conception*. Boston: Beacon Press, 1987.

Levine Slover, Sandra. "Third Party Conception: The Ambivalent Solution." Ottawa: *Infertility Awareness* 5, no. 6 (July/August, 1989), Infertility Awareness Association of Canada.

Marrs, Richard P., M.D., and Serono Symposia, USA. *In Vitro Fertilization and Embryo Replacement*. Norwell, MA.: Serona Symposia, USA.

Mattes, Jane. "Should Donor Insemination Information Be More Available?" New York, NY.: *Single Mothers by Choice* 44 (March 1993).

Mickleburgh, Rod. "Fertility Programs Attacked in Study: 'Very Alarming' AIDS Risk Cited." The *Globe and Mail*, 28 April 1993.

"New applications in Assisted Reproductive Technology: Donor Eggs." Toronto: Information paper, The Toronto Hospital.

Rosenthal, M. Sara. *The Gynecological Sourcebook*. Los Angeles: Lowell House, 1994.

———. *The Pregnancy Sourcebook*. Los Angeles: Lowell House, 1994.

"Secrecy in DI: The 'Advantages' Are the Disadvantages." Ottawa: Infertility Awareness Association of Canada patient information.

"The Sexual Legacy of Infertility: The Separation of Procreation and Recreation." *The Canadian Journal of Human Sexuality* 2, no. 3 (Fall 1993).

"Technological Services for Reproductive Medicine." Toronto: ReproMed Ltd. client information.

Toledo, Andrew A., Micheal J. Tucker, James K. Bennett, Bruce G. Green, Hilton I. Kort, Sharon R. Wiker, and Graham Wright. "Electroejaculation in Combination with In Vitro Fertilization and Gamete Micromanipulation of Anejaculatory Male Infertility." *American Journal of Obstetrics and Gynecology*, August 1992.

Tucker, Michael J., Sharon R. Wiker, Graham Wright, Paula C. Morton, and Andrew Toledo. "Treatment of Male Infertility and Idiopathic Failure to Fertilizie In Vitro with Under Zona Insemination and Direct Egg Injection." *American Journal of Obsttrics and Gynecology*, August 1993.

Van Steirteghem, André C., Jiaen Liu, Hubert Joris, Zsolt Nagy, Cécile Janssenwillen, Herman Tournaye, Marie-Paule Derde, Elvire Van Assche and Paul Devroey. "Higher Success Rate by Intracytoplsmic Sperm Injection Than by Subzonal Insemination. Report of a Second Series of 300 Consecutive Treatment Cycles." *Human Reproduction* 8, no. 7 (1993): 1055–1060.

Zolbrod, Aline. "The Emotional Distress of the Artificial Insemination Patient. *Medical Psychotherapy* 1 (1988): 161–172.

Chapter 9

Carson, Sandra A., and John E. Buster. "Ectopic Pregnancy." *The New England Journal of Medicine* 329 (October 14, 1993).

"Depressive Symptoms after Miscarriage (Tips from Other Journals)." *American Family Physician* 45 (June 1992).

Drife, James Owen. "Tubal Pregnancy: Rising Incidence, Earlier Diagnosis, More Conservative Treatment." *British Medical Journal* 301 (November 10, 1990).

"Early Detection of Ectopic Pregnancy: Use of a Sensitive Urine Pregnancy Test and Transvaginal Ultrasonography." *Journal of the American Medical Association* 266 (November. 13, 1991).

Rosenfeld, Jo Ann. "Bereavement and Grieving after Spontaneous Abortion." *American Family Physician* 43 (May 1991).

Rosenthal, M. Sara. *The Pregnancy Sourcebook*. Los Angeles: Lowell House, 1994.

"Significance of Bleeding During First Trimester (Tips From Other Journals)" *American Family Physician* 44 (November 1991).

"Tubal Pregnancies: Casualty of the Modern Lifestyle." *The Women's Letter* 4 (February 1991).

"Use of Ultrasonography to Diagnose Ectopic Pregnancy (Tips From Other Journals)." *American Family Physician* 42 (November 1990).

Chapter 10

"Adoption in the People's Republic of China." Ottawa: Infertility Awareness Association of Canada factsheet.

"Are You Interested in Adopting from China, Peru, El Salvador, China, Guatemala, Poland, or Bulgaria?" Ottawa: Infertility Awareness Association of Canada factsheet.

Chihal, H. Jane, M.D., and Sister Mary Madonna Baudier, M.D. "Polycystic Ovary Syndrome." *American Family Physician*, April 1985.

"Childless and Second Class." Ottawa: Infertility Awareness Association of Canada factsheet, 1994.

Cunningham, Laura. "The Chosen One." *Hers* magazine, April 17, 1994.

European Adoption Consultants. North Royalton, Ohio: Client information.

Family Focus Adoption Services. Little Neck, New York: client information.

"Friends in Adoption." Middletown Springs, Vermont: Friends in Adoption, Inc. client information.

Galceso, Angela. Welland, Ontario: International Adoption Facilitator client information.

Herman, Flory G. "Private Adoption." Williamsville, New York: attorney client information.

Independent Adoption Centres. Client information.

International Adoption Consultants. Grand Rapids, Michigan: client information.

"Openness in Adoption." Kingston, Ontario: Adoption Resource and Counselling Services.

Radis, David J. Los Angeles: attorney client information.

Raphael, Larry. Chicago: attorney client information.

General Texts

DeMarco, Carolyn. *Take Charge of Your Body: A Woman's Guide to Health*. Winlaw B.C.: The Last Laugh, 1990.

Gorman, Christine. "How Old is Too Old?" *Time*, September 30, 1991.

Harkness, Carla. *The Infertility Book: A Comprehensive Medical and Emotional Guide*. San Francisco: Volcano Press, 1987.

Hey, Valerie, Catherine Itzin, Lesley Saunders, and Mary Anne Speakman, eds. *Hidden Loss: Miscarriage and Ectopic Pregnancy*, London: The Women's Press Ltd., 1989.

Jones, Deborah. "Recurrent Miscarriages: News About Causes and Treatments." *Chatelaine* magazine, November, 1993.

Mullens, Anne. *Missed Conceptions: Overcoming Infertility*. New York: McGraw-Hill, 1990.

Pullen, Heather, and Jocelyn Smith. *Making Babies: A Complete Guide to Fertility and Infertility*. New York: Random House, 1990.

Raab, Diana. *Getting Pregnant and Staying Pregnant: A Guide to Infertility and High-Risk Pregnancy*. Montreal: Sirdan Publishing, 1987.

Seibel, Machelle, M., M.D. *Infertility*. Norwalk, Connecticut: Appleton and Lange, 1990.

Appendix
Where to Go for More Information

The following organizations can provide you with lists of appropriate specialists, fertility clinics in your area, and facilities that can provide you with donor materials. The United States and Canada are listed separately. A list of adoption facilities for both the United States and Canada is also provided.

United States

Adoption
Adoptive Families of America
3333 Highway 100 North
Minneapolis, MN 55422
(612) 535-4829

Concerned United Birthparents
   (CUB)
2000 Walker Street
Des Moines, IA 50317
(515) 262-2334

Cradle of Hope Adoption Center,
   Inc.
1815 H Street N.W.
Suite 1050
Washington D.C. 20006
(202) 296-4700
Fax (202) 785-8131

International Adoption Consultants
1901 Sylvan S.E.
Grand Rapids, MI 49506
(616) 452-1910

National Adoption Information
   Clearinghouse
11426 Rockville Pike
Rockville, MD 20852
(301) 231-6512

New Families, Inc.
15959 S.W. 172 Avenue
Miami, Florida 33187
(305) 254-8425
Fax (305) 238-6789

North American Council on Adopt-
   able Children
970 Raymond Avenue, Suite 106
St. Paul, MN 55391
(612) 473-9372

General
American College of Obstetrics
   and Gynecology (ACOG)
600 Maryland Avenue, S.W.,
   Suite 300
Washington, D.C., 20024
(202) 638-5577

American Fertility Society (AFS)
2140 11th Avenue South, Suite 200
Birmingham, AL 35205–2800
(205) 933-8494

Fertility Research Foundation
877 Park Avenue
New York, NY 10021
(212) 744-5500

Mind/Body Medical Institute
Harvard Medical School
New England Deaconess Hospital
185 Pilgrim Road
Boston, MA, 02215
(617) 623-9525
Fax 617-632-7383

Natural Healing for Infertility
Aline P. Zoldbrod, Ph.D.,
   psychologist
12 Rumford Road
Lexington, Massachusetts 02173
(617) 863-1877

Resolve, Inc.
1310 Broadway
Somerville, MA 02144-1731
Help line: (617) 623-0744
Business office: (617) 623-1156

Serono Symposia USA
100 Longwater Circle
Norwell, MA 02061
(800) 283-8088

DES
The DES Cancer Network
DES Action USA
1615 Broadway
Oakland, CA 94612
(510) 465-4011

Endometriosis
Endometriosis Association
8585 North 76th Place
Milwaukee, WI 53223
(800) 992-3636

Endometriosis Network
Toronto Information Line
(416) 591-3963

St. Charles Medical Centre
Endometriosis Treatment Program
2500 NE Neff Road
Bend, OR 97701
(800) 446-2177

Childfree Living
The Childfree Network
777 Sunset Boulevard, Suite 1800
Citrus Heights, CA 95610
(916) 773-7178

Childless By Choice (CBC)
P.O. Box 695
Leavenworth, WA 98826
(509) 763-2112

NO KIDDING!
Box 27001
Vancouver, British Columbia,
    Canada V5R 6A8
(604) 538-7736

Canada

Adoption

Adoption Agency and Counselling
    Service (Ontario)
Head Office
2349 Fairview Street, Suite 107
Burlington, Ontario, Canada
(416) 507-4037

Adoption Council of Canada
Box 8442, Station T.
Ottawa, Canada K1G 3H8
(613) 235-1566

Adoption Council of Ontario
134 Clifton Road
Toronto, Ontario, Canada M4T 2G6
(416) 482-0021
Fax 416-484-7454

Adoption Helper
189 Springdale Boulevard
Toronto, Ontario, Canada M4C 1Z6
(416) 463-9412

The Adoption Unit
Ministry of Community and
    Social Services
2 Bloor Street West, 24th Floor
Toronto, Ontario, Canada
    M7A 1E9
(416) 327-4730

Canadian Homes for Russian
    Children
1183 Finch Avenue West, #609
North York, Ontario, Canada
    M3J 2G2
(416) 667-7666
Fax (416) 667-7679

Children's Aid Society of
    Metropolitan Toronto
Adoption Services
33 Charles Street
Toronto, Ontario, Canada M4Y 1R9
(416) 924-4646

Children's Institute/Instituto de
    Ninos
220 Cambria Street
Stratford, Ontario, Canada M5A 1J1
(519) 273-7121

Children's Resource and Consulta-
    tion Centre of Ontario
25 Imperial Street, Suite 300
Toronto, Ontario, Canada M5P 1B9
(416) 488-7700
Fax (416) 488-7715

Families in Adoption
134 Clifton Road
Toronto, Ontario, Canada M4T 2G6
(416) 487-9938

International Adoption Services
68 Leaside Drive
Welland, Ontario, Canada L3C 6B2
(905) 732-1643

Jewels for Jesus Adoption Agency
6981 Millcreek Drive, Unit #22
Mississauga, Ontario, Canada
    L5N 6B8
(416) 821-7494

LAAF (Latin American Adoptive
    Families) in Canada
2250 Heidi Avenue
Burlington, Ontario, Canada
    L7M 3W4
(416) 332-3621

The Open Door Society of Ottawa
P.O. Box 9141, Station T
Ottawa, Ontario, Canada K1G 3T8

Single Parent Adoption Support
    Group
40 Riverdale Avenue
Toronto, Ontario, Canada M4K 1C3
(416) 469-2424

SPARK: (Support for Parents
    Adopting Romanian Kids)
19 Knotty Pine Trail
Thornhill, Ontario, Canada
    L3T 3W5
(416) 731-1350

TDH-Canada (Terre des Hommes-
    Canada)
10 St. Mary Street, Suite 506
Toronto, Ontario, Canada
(416) 966-9003
Fax (416) 924-9889

TDH-Canada Montreal office
2520 Lionel Groulx, Suite 5
Montreal, Canada H3J 1J8

General

Association Québécoise pour la Fer-
    tilité Inc.
8000 Boulevard Langelier, Suite 804
St. Leonard, Quebec, Canada
    H1P 3K7

DES Action Canada
P.O. Box 233
Snowdon, Montreal, Quebec
    H3X 3T4
(514) 482-3204

Infertility Awareness Association of
    Canada (IAAC)
104-1785 Vista Drive
Ottawa, Ontario, Canada, Canada
    K1G 3Y6
(613) 738-8968
Fax:(613) 738-0159

IVF Canada
2347 Kennedy Road, Suite 304
Scarborough, Ontario, Canada
    M1T 3T8
(416) 754-8742

Serena Canada
151 Holland Avenue
Ottawa, Ontario, Canada K1Y 0Y2
(613) 728-6536

Index